DEE-TROIT DIET

BY BILL LAITNER

Published by the Detroit Free Press
321 W. Lafayette Blvd.
Detroit, Michigan 48231

© Detroit Free Press Inc., 1989

Cover design by Wayne Kamidoi

Printed by Gaylord Printing Company, Detroit, Michigan

Manufactured in the United States of America

ISBN 0-937247-15-4

I

Acknowledgments

This book and the newspaper articles on which it was based would not have been possible without the assistance of many persons, both inside and outside of the Detroit Free Press organization.

First, I am indebted to Dr. Charles Lucas and his staff at the Beaumont Hospital Clinics of Preventive and Nutritional Medicine, based in Birmingham, Mich.

Dr. Lucas is well known for his outstanding research on obesity, cholesterol, diabetes and other weight-related subjects, and for his success in helping patients with severe weight problems. Dee-troit Diet articles have benefited from four years of his authoritative help, always given with a smile despite his extremely busy schedule. I admire him as a researcher, caring doctor and outstanding marathon runner who absolutely practices what he preaches, and I'm honored that he has written an important foreword to this book.

After my first interviews with Dr. Lucas, I soon began getting expert help from his staff of dietitians and nutritionists, including dietitian Ginnie Uhley, whose research is cited in the pages that follow; nurse-nutritionist Leslie Carroll-Michals, whose advice on menus and recipes has been invaluable; registered dietitian Kristin Miller and dietitian Kathy Clark, who helped in numerous ways.

Many others have been very helpful, among them: Michael Zemel, PhD, a nutrition researcher at Wayne State University in Detroit; Carl Karoub, MD, a preventive medicine specialist at William Beaumont Hospital, Royal Oak, Mich.; and Adam Drewnowski, PhD, an obesity researcher at the University of Michigan, Ann Arbor.

I also owe thanks to many editors at the Free Press, both those who helped make the original articles happen and those who supported me in whipping this book into digestible form: to Scott Bosley and Kathy O'Gorman, who helped with the earliest concepts; to Alice George and Ken Clover, who assisted in conceiving this book; to a superb Free Press book production team that included distribution coordinators Marsha Banks and Thelma Oakes, cover production staff Ken Elenich and Ben Navarro, cover photographer Richard Lee, illustrator Moses Harris, copy editor Barb Arrigo, and designers Wayne Kamidoi, Luis Rios and Lee Yarosh; and to Ann Olson and Michael P. Smith, whose suggestions and careful editing made a difference. Smith was the principal editor of this book; for his diligence I will always be grateful.

And a special thanks goes to my wife, Diana, for countless hours of shopping, cooking, recipe testing, tasting, improving and innovating. Many of "my" best ideas were hers.

Finally, thanks should go to all the readers of the Free Press who, over the last four years, have inspired and informed me with phone calls and letters (from as far away as Australia!). They've shared their diet trials and triumphs on the way to slimmer, healthier lives.

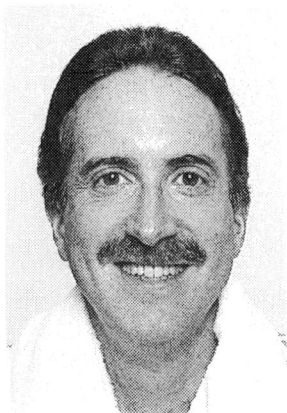

Bill Laitner
Health and Fitness Writer
Detroit Free Press

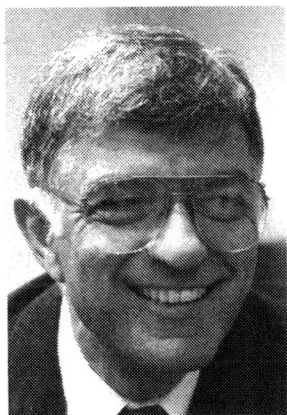

Dr. Charles P. Lucas, M.D., F.A.C.P.
Chief, Division of Preventive and Nutritional Medicine
William Beaumont Hospital
Royal Oak and Birmingham, Michigan

Table of Contents

Chapter 1

Basic Principles of the Dee-troit Diet: Why It Works

Chapter 2

Basic Rules of the Dee-troit Diet: How It Works

Chapter 3

Winning the Numbers Game:
Don't Cut Calories, Cut FAT Calories!

Chapter 4

How to Spy Fat Traps ... in Food and in Yourself

Chapter 5

Anyone's Exercise Plan: It Really Does Burn Off Fat

Chapter 6

Week I of the Dee-troit Diet

Chapter 7

Week II of the Dee-troit Diet

Chapter 8

Week III of the Dee-troit Diet

Chapter 9

Week IV of the Dee-troit Diet

Appendix I: Substitute Breakfasts

Appendix II: For more information . . .

Foreword

By Dr. Charles P. Lucas, M.D., Fellow of the American College of Physicians; and Chief of the Division of Preventive and Nutritional Medicine, at William Beaumont Hospital and affiliated clinics, in Royal Oak, Birmingham, Troy and West Bloomfield, Michigan.

O besity is currently recognized as an important risk factor for heart disease, and for related chronic health problems such as high blood pressure, diabetes and high cholesterol, which contribute to this killer of half a million Americans each year.
     It is of special interest that weight reduction is effective in lowering blood pressure, improving diabetes and correcting the elevated serum cholesterol. Moreover, insurance statistics have shown that policy holders who lose weight during the period of their insurance coverage have a lower death rate from heart attacks than those policy holders who do not lose weight.

In spite of these formidable statistics, the average overweight person is more likely to lose weight in order to better fit into a size 12 dress or a size 40 suit.

Irrespective of the reason people give for wanting to lose weight, the first step in providing an effective therapeutic plan is to understand the critical causes of obesity.

Recent research indicates that the obese have a greater genetic susceptibility to gain weight and a greater tendency to preserve their body fat stores. As a result, when confronted with certain environmental factors — improper diet and physical inactivity — the obese person, as opposed to his or her non-obese counterpart, gains weight.

Successful treatment of obesity can't change genetic susceptibility. However, by selecting a lifelong diet and exercise pattern, the overweight can promote weight loss and weight maintenance, as evidenced by the many successfully treated patients we have observed over the years.

This book by Bill Laitner offers a unique dietary approach that I believe will help you lose weight and maintain your weight loss. Many of the concepts and recipes described in the pages that follow were developed by the nutrition staff of our clinic, who have used this information over the years to produce and maintain weight loss in our moderately obese patients and to minimize weight gain in those with severe obesity who have lost weight on very low-calorie diets.

If you are interested in a diet that also can help lower your cholesterol and blood pressure, can minimize the likelihood of diabetes and heart disease, and still be an enjoyable way of eating for the rest of your life, you will find useful information in this book.

Importantly, this diet also meets the following criteria: It is nutritionally sound; it supplies the optimal daily requirements for protein, fiber, minerals, vitamins and essential fatty acids; it is low in caloric density; it is low in fat; and it has enough flavor and texture so that one can follow it for a lifetime.

All of these factors make it ideal for weight reduction, weight maintenance, and long-term compliance.

Introduction

Where did the Dee-troit Diet come from? Who originated it, and what makes it different from the scores of other diet and nutrition books intended for the public?

This book grew out of more than 40 articles published in the Detroit Free Press from 1986 through 1989. These articles provided a weight-loss plan that appeared in the form of seven separate weeks of diet stories.

Through the resources of the Knight Ridder Tribune News service, many of the articles were published in other newspapers under the name "The Seven Day Diet" — because each segment was one week long.

Thus, not just Detroit Free Press readers have been Dee-troit Dieting. So have readers of the New York Daily News, and those of newspapers from Buffalo, N.Y., to Biloxi, Miss., with Charleston, S.C., and others in between.

Here's how the diet came to be and what makes it different . . .

As health and fitness columnist at the Free Press, I had written numerous articles on nutrition, weight loss, exercise and health before sitting down with editors to plan the first Dee-troit Diet series. When

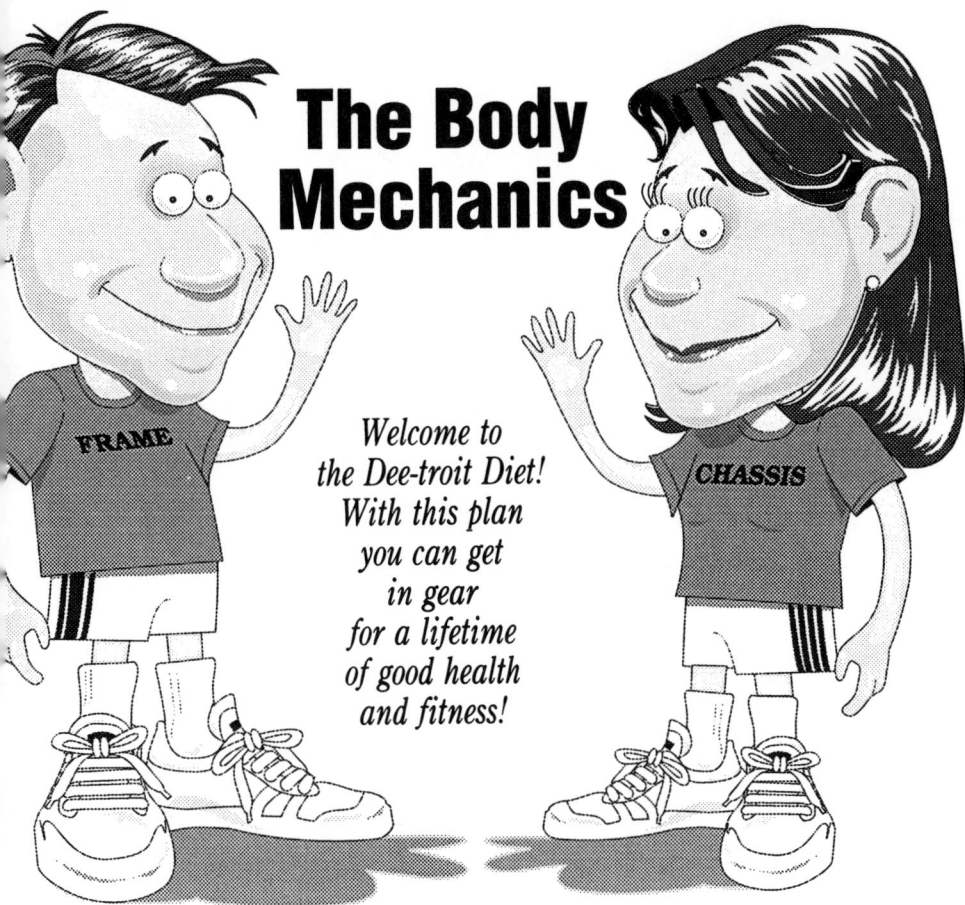

The Body Mechanics

*Welcome to
the Dee-troit Diet!
With this plan
you can get
in gear
for a lifetime
of good health
and fitness!*

FRAME

CHASSIS

that first week of Dee-troit Dieting ended, it was clear that our series had received a far greater response from readers than previous health articles.

Evidently, there was a big appetite for plain, newspaper-style talk on healthful food and sensible dieting.

At first, that surprised us, because we at the Free Press had thought the weight-loss market was saturated. Indeed, the flood of diet books has been steady through the 1980s. Publishers worldwide vie for attention with bolder claims and gaudier press releases. Some even send food!

Yet despite the slick promotion of most diet books in stores and on

TV talk shows, it became evident that publishers were missing a sizable market. Despite celebrity endorsements on dust covers, imposing credentials of doctors with prominent practices in Manhattan or Beverly Hills, catchy names of many diets — many diet books were missing the mark with Free Press readers here in Middle America.

"Comin' up! One down-to-earth diet plan."

Southeast Michigan is the Motor Capital of the World, birthplace of the car and assembly line. Here, livelihoods are less likely to spring from East Coast-style financial wizardry or Hollywood-style glitz. Detroit's style evolved from old-fashioned sweat combined with American ingenuity.

As you might expect, then, readers of the Detroit Free Press tend to be a down-to-earth, home lovin' group. They're not much inclined to embrace imports like the Scarsdale Diet, the Beverly Hills Diet and the Southampton Diet. This isn't a town that wants to downsize on Japanese mushrooms, Scandinavian flatbread, or French goat cheese and champagne.

So what's this about "Dee-troit"? Among friends, longtime Detroiters sometimes pronounce the old town's name the way they first heard it, or their grandfathers did. They say *"Dee-*troit," accenting that first syllable.

And so, the idea for the Dee-troit Diet was born. At the Free Press, we felt it was time for an unhyped, unpretentious, homegrown diet plan.

Banned would be exotic foods, unusual claims, narrow theories, and expensive and unnecessary regimens of vitamins or other supplements. We wanted the Dee-troit Diet to offer straightforward transportation. We wanted whatever would get us safely and efficiently to our readers' goals, namely, permanent weight loss and better health.

First, we needed a diet designer . . .

Happily, we found the perfect source for research data, for clinical experience with a wide range of overweight patients, and for tasty recipes and tested menus, and we found that source right here in our midst. Charles Lucas, M.D., and his staff of obesity researchers and clinicians were quietly perfecting their obesity-fighting program at Detroit's Wayne State University, using common sense backed by state-of-the-art research, their own as well as a growing consensus from other research sites.

It was Dr. Lucas (who has since moved his expanded practice to suburban Detroit) — along with his large staff of nutritionists, dietitians, exercise physiologists and behavioral psychologists — who helped us fashion the original Dee-troit Diet articles on which this book is based.

Then, readers tried the first diet menus . . .

Reader response to the early stories was exciting. More than 6,000 readers requested reprints of the first diet installments. Of course, our handsome Dee-troit Diet T-shirts were gone in a flash that year.

Surprisingly, a fellow from the land of movies and posh fat farms got the very last T-shirt. It happened when Dee-troit Diet fans told us they'd watched Bob Hope's "All-Star Super Bowl Party," broadcast in January 1986. Hope, in a skit with oversized football pro William (The Refrigerator) Perry, kidded him about his size and said, "Hey, did you hear about the new Detroit Diet? As soon as you eat a meal, it's recalled."

Hope's publicist later confirmed that Hope's writers had heard about the Free Press series. At that publicist's request, we sent Hope the very last Dee-troit Diet T-shirt.

It turns out that our timing is almost as good as Hope's. The Dee-troit Diet arrived just as major health organizations, like the American Heart Association and American Cancer Society, were reaching a consensus with athletes, weight-loss specialists and experts in heart disease, cancer and other diseases. It turns out that a common nutritional approach has become the acknowledged route to slimness *and* better health *and* top athletic performance.

So, no fad foods or diet secrets here . . .

The Dee-troit Diet is just a common-sense approach that works. It uses the low-fat principles that all major health groups now endorse. Then, we make it as easy, convenient, tasty and flexible as we possibly can.

We've collected the best recipes from four years of Free Press diet articles, expanding the sections that help explain the diet and motivate you to eat right and exercise. At the same time, we've included numerous frozen dinner and microwave options, even many fast-food and chain restaurant selections.

Our recipe theme? Middle American, of course. Increasing numbers of Americans, and many posh restaurants as well, are turning away from fussy, imported, high-fat delicacies. We're returning to the traditional food many of us grew up with, the family-style recipes that are often called "comfort food."

That's the basis of what you'll find here: Low-fat, easy-to-make versions of traditional favorites, adapted to fit the latest but widely acknowledged principles of low-fat, high-fiber nutrition, with additional emphasis on food that helps improve blood cholesterol levels. These are recipes and menus you can keep using, long after you've reached your target weight, to look and feel your best.

And so we hope this expanded Dee-troit Diet, and the accompanying exercise plan, get you where you want to go — looking slimmer and feeling better than ever.

1

Basic Principles of the Dee-troit Diet: Why It Works

W elcome to the Dee-troit Diet, the beginning of a journey to a slimmer, healthier you. We hope our diet and exercise plan is something you'll try.

And not just for a week or two. Because even though we suggest specific meal plans to follow, we're not saying to stop when you're done reading.

Instead, this book can be the beginning of lifetime changes in your eating habits.

Of course, no single book can answer every nutrition question and need. But we think this slim volume offers a bite-sized, good-tasting start to what can be a lifetime of more sensible eating and exercising, not to mention a skinnier you.

You will find no amazing claims here, no "secret" research findings revealed, no single diet food that "melts off pounds," no one-minute-a-day exercise "breakthroughs" that lose inches instantly. Neither is there any exotic and costly food called for in our recipes, nor any vitamin megadoses requiring repeated treks to health food stores. Everything you need can be purchased in your local supermarket, in some cases even your nearby fast-food restaurant!

This book can be your first step to getting off the roller coaster of special fad diets. Far too often, they revolve around a single food, such as rice, grapefruit or popcorn. Or they claim a breakthrough with a single concept or behavior pattern, like eating more on some days and less on others. Worst of all, far too many of these diet plans approach weight control and healthful eating as a temporary fix, something to be endured for "X" number of weeks, after which the "dieter" again becomes a normal non-dieting American, returning quickly to the typical intake of about 40 percent fat calories.

This book is aimed at starting you on a realistic improvement in your permanent quality of nutritional life. Yes, the emphasis is on *quality*, not quantity. Even though this book spells out a reduced-calorie plan, for helping you achieve a target weight, and even though we think the ideas and recipes here will help you achieve that target, our ultimate goal is not to cut the quantity of food you eat. Improving the *quality* of your diet is what we're after.

Eat as much as you want?

Yes, you can have just about as much as you want of the right foods, once you've made the transition to a high-quality diet. We'll show you how to do it by weaning you off fat and onto lean, fresh, exciting taste experiences, without sacrificing convenience or your budget.

After you've tried our recipes, we'll point you toward some of the best sources of other recipes that fulfill the basic Dee-troit Diet principles. You'll find that our diet and exercise plan, instead of claiming to be a breakthrough or radical departure, is instead at the very center of a mainstream revolution in America's nutritional thinking. We've simply chosen some winning recipes with a track record of success among truly obese individuals. Then we've fine-tuned the best new information to make it as easy as possible to understand, to reach your goals, and to incorporate sensible eating and exercise into the rest of your life.

We do it with a low-fat diet that is high in complex carbohydrates. These are the fresh fruits, vegetables and whole-grain foods that have become the widely accepted choices of everyone from Olympic athletes to cardiologists, preventive cancer experts and obesity specialists. We also use mild levels of the sustained, fat-burning exercise that doctors call "aerobic" (more strenuous activity is optional). Aerobic exercise is the type that's best for everyone from diabetics, heart patients and obese individuals to endurance athletes and everyday, ordinary, slightly over-weight people.

What the Dee-troit Diet can do for you

■ First, we slim you down.

Losing weight is just about everyone's goal. But our diet and exercise plan helps you lose *fat,* at a doctor-approved rate of one to two pounds a week.

We'll show you low-fat menus and recipes to start you on a path that our diet designers — a top obesity researcher and his staff of nutritionists and behavioral psychologists — have used to help thousands of patients make permanent changes to good eating habits, not merely achieve temporary weight losses.

*Basic
Principles
of the
Dee-troit
Diet: Why
It Works*

On the Dee-troit Diet, you'll avoid the fatigue, potential health problems and self-defeating aspects of unbalanced, unsupervised crash dieting.

It's true that very low-calorie diets can work for seriously obese patients, if they are supervised by doctors and other obesity specialists. Such specialists use liquid diet formulas designed to minimize loss of muscle tissue, and they make sure that patients receive behavior modification counseling and get on exercise programs before returning to healthful, low-fat eating plans like the Dee-troit Diet.

A doctor-supervised very low-calorie diet — sometimes called a protein-sparing modified fast — is safe when "properly administered in an appropriate clinical or outpatient setting," says a 1989 statement by the American Dietetic Association, a group of more than 60,000 nutrition professionals.

But unbalanced, unsupervised crash dieting can sabotage your best intentions. Over several days, it results mostly in the loss of "water weight" instead of fat. Over longer periods, it can lead to more serious problems, including regaining more weight than you lost. Here's why:

When you cut calories too much, your body flicks a switch, so to speak, and quickly learns to survive on less food. In this way, the same mechanism that enabled humans to survive famines can booby-trap your diet. Despite eating less, you may lose relatively little weight. When you return to a normal caloric intake, watch out! The pounds will stick like glue, thanks to your new, lower rate of metabolism — what researchers call "increased feeding efficiency."

This is why many unsupervised crash dieters end up regaining weight more quickly than they lost it, the result of the dreaded but all-too-common "yo-yo syndrome."

Worst of all, dieters who repeat this cycle often regain more weight than they lost.

At the same time, diets of unbalanced, unsupervised starvation rations can jeopardize your health by shorting you on essential nutrients like calcium, iron and fiber. The same problem often occurs with popular fad or celebrity diets, which tend to concentrate on one food or one nutritional concept, to the exclusion of a balanced diet. And those who pop vitamins, minerals and other nutrients in place of nutritious food are kidding themselves. Most nutritionists and dietitians agree: Supplements are no substitute for getting the right nutrition, in balanced amounts, from good food.

■ **Second, we improve your health.**

You see, Dee-troit Dieting does much more than slim you down. It will help lower your cholesterol level, by minimizing foods containing cholesterol and fat, particularly saturated fat. We've also included food that actually helps remove cholesterol from your body or provide other protective factors against heart disease.

The Dee-troit Diet will probably cut your sodium intake, too, if you consume salt the way most Americans do. And it will fight symptoms of dietary deficiencies with inexpensive food loaded with calcium, iron, fiber and other nutrients. If you're concerned about osteoporosis, for example, you'll be glad to know that this diet is high in calcium.

The Dee-troit Diet is also chock full of fiber, what some people call roughage. That's the stuff scientists say everybody needs more of, to fight everything from hemorrhoids to cancer.

Besides making you healthier and thinner, Dee-troit Dieting may very well give you more energy. That's because the diet's nutrient principles are similar to those of the training tables of major endurance-sport champions, including top finishers of the Ironman Triathlon in Hawaii and the Detroit Free Press International Marathon.

Foods on the diet are also on the training table of marathoner Dr. Charles Lucas, M.D., our Dee-troit Diet designer. He's a nationally known obesity researcher, university lecturer, and director of a major Detroit-area hospital's weight-loss program (the Beaumont Clinics of Preventive and Nutritional Medicine, based in Birmingham). Lucas and his staff of nutritionists and behavioral psychologists have helped hundreds of severely overweight patients lose thousands of pounds of unattractive, unhealthy excess weight. One patient started out weighing more than a quarter of a ton!

We've put together the Dee-troit Diet based on their clinical experience. We've tested and fine-tuned their best recipes and diet ideas, then added many of our own.

Now, read on for a quick summary of basic Dee-troit Diet principles.

The fat facts of life

■ **Eating fat makes you fat!**

Remember that line. It's the single most important principle behind the Dee-troit Diet.

If you have a serious relationship with fatty foods, we're *soooo* sorry. We'll be helping you break off the affair, something you'll thank us for as soon as you find out how much better you look and feel.

Granted, there are lots of things that contribute to being overweight. Among them are inactivity, eating too many total calories, and hereditary dispositions to a low metabolism rate and to obesity itself.

Still, for most Americans, the bottom line on waistlines is simply that *eating fat makes us fat.* That's been the finding of many major research studies with both humans and animals.[1] And it's the clear conclusion and favorite saying of Dr. Charles Lucas, our Dee-troit Diet designer.

There are several reasons. For one thing, fat is the most concentrated source of calories. A single gram of fat has double the calories of a gram of carbohydrate or protein. That means that high-fat foods — from cheeseburgers to chocolate bars, from steak to salad dressing, whole milk to whole eggs — are crammed with densely packed calories.

"So by simply cutting out a few fat foods, you're going to cut back significantly on calories," says Dr. Lucas.

Another key point? Even when fat eaters count their calories, they seem to put on the pounds. Studies of rats show that "1,000 calories of fat makes a fatter rat than 1,000 calories of carbohydrates," says Lucas. The reason is that rats (and humans) use many more times the energy to digest and store carbohydrates than they (and humans) do to store fats. That means people work off weight just by digesting an apple or a plain baked potato; but a pat of butter slides down the hatch and onto the waistline almost effortlessly!

■ **Eating fat triggers the yo-yo effect**

The rats in obesity experiments must know that discouraged feeling. Take the research trials overseen by a Lucas clinic staff member, head dietitian Ginnie Uhley. At Detroit's Wayne State University, she put a pack of rats on a preliminary period of weight reduction, then set up one brood on a high-fat diet, another on a low-fat regimen.

Says Uhley: "The ones on the high-fat diet actually took in fewer calories, but they were able to gain more weight. In fact, after the initial weight loss, they immediately went back to their original weights and then continued to go *higher.*"

Sound familiar? Even rats can become yo-yos in the body fat game.

The nation's high-fat diet helps explain why the percentage of overweight Americans today is five to eight times greater than in 1900. Not only are modern Americans less active than their ancestors were at the turn of the century, but also they eat about 30 percent more fat

Basic Principles of the Dee-troit Diet: Why It Works

despite a *decrease* in the total calories they eat.

For all of the above reasons, and more, the key component of the Dee-troit Diet is reduced fat intake. The rest of the story, in a nutshell? It's reduced cholesterol intake as well.

We've crowded out fat and cholesterol with heaps of complex carbohydrates, nature's best energy source. They're found in whole grains, fruits and vegetables.

■ Eating fat makes you hungry

Fat foods, because they are dense, can be eaten quickly. Yet they don't fill you up. So you want more just to feel satisfied. And let's face it, how you feel during and after eating is very important.

"If you could pack 1,000 calories into a thimble, I'm sure people would find a way to eat 10,000 calories a day," says Dr. Lucas.

Carbohydrate foods provide the very opposite effect.

"You fill up faster on carbohydrate foods, which are bulkier, so you feel fuller on fewer calories," says dietitian Ginnie Uhley.

As far as moods go, research at the Massachusetts Institute of Technology suggests that a high-fat meal makes you more sluggish and less alert, although scientists aren't sure why.

What is proven is that fat molecules can act something like appetite triggers. They're excellent at transporting intense flavors, then helping those flavors remain in the mouth as tempting after-tastes. They even provide a special sensation all their own, called "mouth feel."

That means your food plan needs some fats to create delectable recipes, the kind both dieters and family members who *aren't* dieting will enjoy. It also means that you'll need to portion out those fats, distributing them at meals, and carefully avoiding them between meals when they may act as triggers to temptation.

■ Fat makes you unhealthy

Almost everyone agrees. Just ask traditional health groups like the American Heart Association, American Cancer Society and the Arthritis Foundation; or the acres of researchers in Uncle Sam's National Institutes of Health; and the author of just about any recent book on nutrition, or the clerk behind the counter of a typical health food store.

The excess fat Americans eat along with the excess fat stored in their bodies combine to become the major contributor to the diet-caused ills of modern America.

Fat promotes heart disease and stroke, cancer, bowel troubles — even constipation and hemorrhoids. Yes, high-fat, processed foods first elbow out of your diet the fiber that aids digestion and excretion, then allow digested food to become so tightly compressed in the colon that the tissue damage of diverticulitis (severely irritated colon) and hemorrhoids can result.

The fat you eat and the fat you store in your body both lead to high levels of cholesterol in the blood, too. That, in turn, leads to heart disease, heart attack and stroke.

What about cutting out high-cholesterol foods? Yes, reducing the intake of *dietary* cholesterol — the cholesterol in food, that is — can indeed help reduce the level of *serum* cholesterol floating around in the bloodstream and clogging arteries. But researchers now believe that the fat in food, particularly the insidious kind called saturated fat, does more to raise blood cholesterol in the typical American than does the cholesterol in food.[2]

Dietary and body fat also promotes numerous kinds of cancer, including that of the breast, colon, uterus, prostate, ovary and pancreas. And fat plays a role in many other diseases. Not the least of them is obesity itself, which in extreme cases becomes a life-threatening disease, often tied to high blood pressure (hypertension) and diabetes (the adult-onset type).

And there are other medical problems, from gallstones to blood-clotting disorders, largely the result of the all-American, high-fat diet.

All this doesn't even mention the *mental health* aspects of being overweight and living on fatty foods. Who can possibly document the epidemic of fatigue, low self-esteem and depression that has resulted from the incessant fattening of America?

■ So . . . how much fat is OK?

Almost none, say nutritional extremists. No more than 30 percent of total calories, says the American Heart Association. A host of others suggest levels in between.

Among major public health groups like the Heart Association, leaders know that if they could just get millions of Americans to cut out a quarter of the fat consumed, dropping daily fat calorie intake to about 30 percent, then as a nation we'd take giant steps toward improved health.

Still, there are many who are close to obesity research, and close to the clinical world of overweight patients, who think that a limit under 30 percent has important benefits.

Signs point to a need to lower fat intake below 30 percent for many Americans with stubbornly high cholesterol levels. And experience shows that when you do, weight loss and other health improvements truly accelerate.

That's why our Dee-troit Diet designers want to slash your fat intake in half. They settled on a fat limit of 15 to 20 percent of total calories, both

1

*Basic
Principles
of the
Dee-troit
Diet: Why
It Works*

for their severely overweight obesity patients, for themselves in everyday meals, and for Dee-troit Dieters. That means once you make the permanent switch in your nutritional habits, you'll be eating less than half the fat of the 40-percent fat diet consumed by Mr. and Ms. Average American.

And to give your body an extra-fast start at shedding fat, most of the Dee-troit Diet menus in this book are even lower. Some are 15 percent fat, some 10 percent, sometimes even less! But we've dropped the numbers only when we could preserve good-tasting meals. You'll be the beneficiary because our diet weeks will accelerate your initial fat loss.

Yet for the most part, the Dee-troit Diet is far from extreme. It's considerably more flexible than ultra-low-fat programs such as the Pritikin Plan. Many of these programs cut fat to 8 percent or even less.

For the vast majority of us, ultra-low-fat diets aren't the answer. They may sound good on paper, since the numbers are attractive to purists. But they just aren't practical, because they aren't tasty enough for most people and they're just about impossible to attain in restaurants or with convenience foods.

Here's what one top nutritional authority, a leading researcher on the tastes people love most and why, says about the Pritikin and other ultra-low-fat diets:

"So much of these meals taste like a sort of gruel. They're just not palatable to the vast majority of Americans." [3]

That same researcher, a University of Michigan professor and director of that institution's Program in Human Nutrition, has determined through research that overeaters are not so much turned on to overindulging by a "sweet tooth" as by a "fat tooth."

That's right: Fat makes you fat, but it is also a primeval signal of taste satisfaction in humans. The reason is, fat molecules transport food flavors better than protein or carbohydrate molecules. Fat molecules also help retain those good tastes on your taste buds, and they provide the satisfying "body" or "mouth feel" of many foods.

Thus, cutting fat to a bare, Pritikin-style minimum takes much of the pleasure out of what should be one of life's more rewarding sensuous delights — namely, eating! It's virtually impossible, not to mention cruel, to expect people to lead deprived lives at mealtimes for the sake of weight loss or improved health.

And guess what? You don't have to. Just read on to learn about the very first Dee-troit Dieters!

The Dee-troit Diet, Stone-Age style

Some assiduous scientific digging has turned up recent evidence that our prehistoric ancestors had a sizable share of fat at mealtimes.

Yet they lived in bodies that were lean and surprisingly disease-free. Studies of fossilized remains show that if Stone Age people were able to survive the rigors of infancy and childhood, they apparently enjoyed excellent health throughout life.

True, our prehistoric forebears were subject to many infectious diseases that modern medicine today protects against with vaccines and antibiotics. But they suffered far less than we do from the "diseases of civilization" — heart disease, cancer, stroke, obesity and many others.

Researchers at two universities, in separate investigations, combined the disciplines of nutrition, anthropology, archaeology and biochemistry, actually studying the fossilized remains of — are you ready for this? — prehistoric latrines. Sounds stinky, but it isn't. Turns out, fossilized human excrement that is rock-hard and roughly 25,000 years old shows that prehistoric man and woman ate bushels of wild plants — the equivalents of today's fresh fruits, vegetables and whole-grain foods — between meals of meat and fish.

What's more, they walked miles and miles carrying this food once they found it, because they couldn't eat it all at once and because they wanted to share it with family members back at the hut. Sounds just like the latest rage in southern California: Fitness walking with chest weights!

The resulting life-style was a prehistoric family whose intake of fat was moderate. They weren't wolfing down fat, but neither were they existing without it.

The same family also ate large amounts of unrefined plant foods that today are called complex carbohydrates (again, those fresh fruits, veggies and whole-grain breads and cereals). They enjoyed lots of natural sources for such nutrients as Vitamin C and calcium. And their daily activity included plenty of vigorous walking, the very kind of continuous exercise that doctors recommend as aerobic exercise.

All this kept Mr. and Ms. Cave Person quite lean, with low blood cholesterol and fewer risk factors for other diseases associated with overweight. [4]

The next four weeks ... and the rest of your life.

For those of you with average health and overweight problems, a

Basic Principles of the Dee-troit Diet: Why It Works

lifetime limit of 15-20 percent fat calories is not extreme. It's a sure bet to keep you slimmer and healthier, yet it still allows you some special treats and an occasional "night on the town."

For the four weeks of Dee-troit Dieting in this book, we've lowered the fat percentage even more than the everyday target of 15-20 percent that we'd like you to shoot for. Even though we included fast-food meals and some special treats, the meal plans average less than 12 percent in fat calories.

Why? Because we want to accelerate your fat loss and show you that truly low-fat eating isn't impossible. We think you'll agree: It's a fast track to the goals, yet it still enables you to enjoy the positive reinforcement of delicious, inexpensive, everyday foods.

So let's get on with Dee-troit Dieting, pronto. You've just finished learning about the basic principles of Dee-troit Dieting: the "whys."

In the next chapter, we'll get down to business. You'll learn the basic rules to achieve those principles: the "hows."

Then, you'll graduate to healthier grocery shopping and home cooking, learning to find hidden sources of fat and how to flush them out by reading labels, especially those on frozen and microwave dinner products. You'll even learn how to find fat disguised in the language of restaurant menus.

Finally, you'll discover some great recipes that'll please the whole family, including members who don't have the slightest weight worry or cholesterol concern.

And on convenience days, you'll find out how something as simple as choosing one frozen microwave dinner over another, or ordering fast-food pizza in a different but delicious way, can save you untold numbers of destructive fat calories, the gremlins that sabotage both your health and appearance.

---

[1] The following two reports in the American Journal of Clinical Nutrition (47:406 and 47:995, 1988) are among many that support the theory that the number of calories you eat isn't as responsible for weight gain or loss as is the number of fat calories:

■ A study from Harvard Medical School looked at 141 women (aged 34-59), and found that, after adjusting for age, physical activity levels, alcohol intake and smoking, there was almost no connection between calorie intake and body weight. There was, however, a strong connection to fat consumption.

■ A study from Stanford University School of Medicine charted eating patterns of 155 sedentary overweight men, aged 30-59, and came to the same conclusion: namely, that body weight was related to fat calories eaten, not to total calories.

[2] Bonnie Liebman, nutrition director, Center for Science in the Public Interest, Washington, D.C.

[3] Adam Drewnowski, PhD, director of the University of Michigan Human Nutrition Program.

[4] See "The Paleolithic Prescription" by Dr. Boyd Eaton, Marjorie Shostak and Melvin Konner (Harper & Row, 1988), all of Emory University; and the research of Vaughn Bryant Jr., professor of anthropology, Texas A&M University.

2

Basic Rules
of the Dee-troit Diet:
How It Works

The Dee-troit Diet emphasis is on improving the *quality* of the food you eat, not cutting the *quantity*.

Thus, crash dieting is *not* allowed. Of course, during the weight-loss phase, you will probably eat somewhat fewer calories than before. But with the addition of filling, bulky, complex carbohydrates, you may find you're even less hungry than before you changed your eating habits. And we'll tell you why there's no reason you should ever feel deprived on the Dee-troit Diet.

How much do you want to weigh?

Your target weight determines roughly how many calories you should eat to foster safe, gradual, permanent weight loss.

For example, let's say you want to weight 120 pounds. Multiply by 10 for your daily calorie count. So, 120 x 10 = 1,200 calories daily.

That's the number of calories we've designed the Dee-troit Diet around. Daily menus, not including two approved snacks per day, total about 1,200 calories, a safe level for achieving a steady weight loss of one to three pounds per week — even more if you exercise — toward a goal weight of 120.

Once you've achieved your goal, you'll find you can eat more calories and still maintain your weight. Typically, the daily amount will be about 11 times your weight in daily calories for women, about 12 times for men. Of course, maintenance amounts vary widely, depending on daily activity levels, especially if you exercise, and on individual metabolism rates. But more about that later.

Budgeted into our plan are two 80-calorie snacks per day, but only from the approved list on Pages 14 and 15. These are foods that contain almost no fat, and their addition of carbohydrate calories won't have a significant effect on your daily calorie target.

You can easily adjust our plan to fit different body sizes, energy needs and weight-loss goals. Just use the formula. Say you want to weigh 128. Multiply your goal weight, 128, by 10. That equals 1,280, and that's the number of calories you need to eat each day to achieve your goal weight.

The Dee-troit Diet in a nutshell

Here's what you'll get on a typical 1,200-calorie day of our weight-loss plan (for those who find this section boring, skip to the next section for getting started on Dee-troit Dieting).

Approximate daily nutrient levels	
Fat	10-15 percent
Carbohydrates	65-70 percent
Protein	20 percent
Cholesterol	less than 100 milligrams (well under the limit suggested by the American Heart Association)
Dietary fiber	more than 25 grams (about twice what most Americans get)
Sodium (salt)	about 1,500 milligrams (less if you make a point of using low-salt ingredients in recipes)
Calcium	about 900 milligrams (more than the Recommended Dietary Allowance for adult women and about twice what the typical American woman gets in her everyday diet)

The diet is also rich in iron, potassium, Vitamins A and C, beta carotene and many other nutrients.

In that case, you'd want to add 80 calories to the Dee-troit Diet menus of 1,200. On Pages 14-15, you'll find a list showing healthful ways to grab an 80-calorie snack. To add more calories, grab more snacks or help yourself to larger portions of our recipe servings. To adjust downward, do the opposite.

If you find yourself feeling deprived or "starved" for whatever reason, grab another one or two of these legal snacks. They're high-quality, low-fat foods that will fill you up with fiber but won't add much if any fat to your diet.

Remember, it's not so much the *quantity* of calories you eat as the *quality* that affects weight, blood cholesterol and general health. Dee-troit Dieters can feel free to eat plenty of the right foods, those low in fat and cholesterol, high in vitamins, fiber and energy — namely, the complex carbohydrates in whole grains, fruits and vegetables.

2

Basic Rules of the Dee-troit Diet: How It Works

Getting started . . .

Now remember, our strategy is two-fold. The two basic plays in our game plan are:

■ We'll wean you off about half of the fat you're probably consuming, replacing it with generous servings of complex carbohydrates, those filling, nutritious fresh fruits, vegetables and whole grains.

You'll probably find yourself eating less protein than before, too, yet not missing it a bit.

■ We'll lower your blood cholesterol with major cutbacks in dietary cholesterol and saturated fat, avoiding egg yolks, red meat, fried food, high-fat dairy products, and tropical oils (coconut, palm and palm kernel).

At the same time, we'll emphasize three food categories beneficial to blood cholesterol levels — the soluble fiber in oat bran, citrus fruit and legumes such as peas; the special oils in fish; and the monounsaturated fats in olive and canola oil.

Sound complicated? It isn't. It'll be as simple as replacing that jar of mayonnaise in your 'fridge with Weight Watchers salad dressing or plain non-fat yogurt. (For added flavor in yogurt "dressing," try mixing just a dab of "light" mayonnaise with the plain yogurt — great on sandwiches!)

The 10 basic rules of Dee-troit Dieting

1. MINIMIZE YOUR FAT INTAKE. Do this by eliminating the following fatty foods: egg yolks (use two egg whites for each whole egg, or use an egg

80-CALORIE

Here are suggestions for Dee-troit Diet snacks. Use these foods, each containing about 80 calories, for adjusting your daily calorie count, by adding snacks to meals or by enjoying them between meals.

Even if you don't need to adjust calories, you're allowed two snacks a day on our 1,200 calorie plan.

■ One slice of bread, preferably whole wheat or other whole-grain type; if desired, spread generously with one tablespoon of low-sugar or artificially sweetened jam or jelly.

■ One-half bagel, preferably whole wheat (plain or garlic bagels are also good; egg bagels are generally too high in fat). Same topping as for bread.

■ Two rice cakes. Same topping as for bread.

■ One half round of pita bread (some people also know this bread from the Middle East as "pocket bread"), preferably whole wheat (five- to six-inch diameter).

■ One cup (8 ounces) of skim milk or three-quarters cup (6 ounces) of plain *non*-fat yogurt (ordinary yogurt, even *low*-fat yogurt, is too high in fat; non-fat yogurt may be eaten plain or flavored with a small amount of low-sugar jam or jelly).

■ One-half cup (4 ounces) of low-fat cottage cheese (no more than 1 percent milk fat).

■ One whole fresh fruit: Your choice, from oranges, grapefruit, bananas, apples and pears to kiwis and kumquats (equivalents include two medium peaches; one cup of grapes, berries, cherries or pineapple chunks). Exclude frozen or canned fruit, especially with added sugar. You can, however, include a fresh, whole tomato — and we won't argue whether it's a fruit or vegetable.

SNACK LIST

For any, you may slice, dress with a tablespoon of lemon juice or store-bought "no oil" dressing (available in supermarkets), and serve on lettuce leaves. Otherwise, simply enjoy plain. And to obtain the special type of fruit fiber that improves cholesterol levels, plan on including several citrus fruits (fresh oranges or grapefruit) each week.

■ One medium plain baked potato, topped with pepper, paprika or butter substitutes such as Butter Buds or Molly McButter, or with a tablespoon of plain non-fat yogurt or a tablespoon of "no-oil" salad dressing (if you order a plain baked potato in a restaurant, especially a fast-food outlet, specify loudly, "No butter on it!").

Note: One of our favorite snacks is letting a baked potato cool in the 'fridge, then eating it right out of hand, sprinkling each bite with a dash of Mrs. Dash Original Flavor Salt-Free seasoning and/or Molly McButter imitation Sour Cream flavor.

■ Two cups of plain popcorn (not packaged microwave products, not even "unbuttered" movie theater popcorn: Both have plenty of fat added in processing). Use the same fat-free buttery toppings as for potatoes; light salt or salt-free seasoning such as Mrs. Dash is optional.

■ One frozen fruit juice bar (such as Dole, Shamitoff, etc.). Only one allowed per day. (Check labels carefully; juice bar maximum is 90 calories and 1 gram of fat per bar.)

■ One Weight Watchers Double Fudge Artificially Flavored Quiescently Frozen Confection (frozen fudge bar), or similar diet dessert item with no more than 90 calories and one gram of fat. Only one allowed per day.

If you need a handy reminder, copy this list and tape it to your refrigerator.

2

*Basic
Rules
of the
Dee-troit
Diet: How
It Works*

10 basic rules:

1. Minimize your fat intake
2. Clean out the junk
3. For cooking, choose monounsaturated fats
4. Switch from fried food
5. Switch from refined, low-fiber carbohydrates
6. Reduce salt intake
7. Eat more fish
8. Reduce your stress level
9. Drink more liquid
10. Exercise

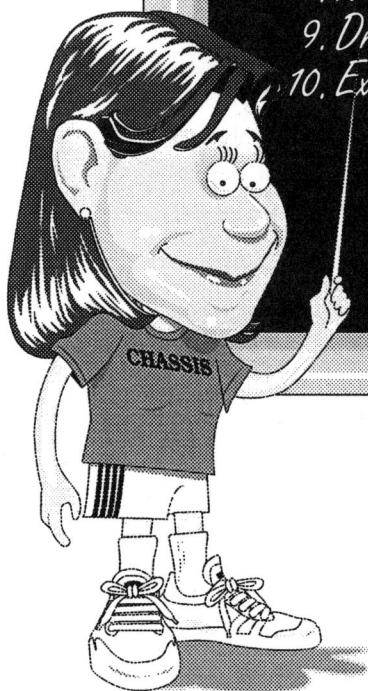

substitute such as Egg Beaters); red meat (instead, eat skinless poultry and fish); cheese (except for low-fat cottage cheese, which contains 1 percent milk fat or less; and modest amounts of part-skim mozzarella, allowed in some recipes); butter, gravy, cream sauces and regular margarine (switch to "light" margarine — the kind that often comes in tubs). Avoid commercial baked goods, most fast-food items, theater popcorn, doughnuts and many frozen dinners.

Instead, use low-fat substitutes, especially for dairy products rich in important calcium. Use powdered butter substitutes, like Butter Buds and Molly McButter, for cooking; non-fat yogurt instead of sour cream; skim milk for whole or 2-percent types; and lemon juice or "no-oil" dressings in place of regular store-bought salad dressing (read labels; look for dressings with less than one gram of fat per tablespoon).

2. CLEAN OUT THE JUNK. Junk food, that is. Ice cream lovers, break off the affair. Clean out freezers and restock with fat-free sherbets and sorbets (Dole makes excellent ones). At the same time, clear out other junk food such as cookies, cakes, candy and high-fat dips. You'll be able to go back to limited portions of a few special treats later, but only after you've achieved your target weight. Having them around now only provides needless temptation.

Do stock your larder with items on our 80-Calorie Snack List. Don't stint. An investment in fresh, wholesome complex carbohydrates is the cheapest health insurance you can buy.

One of the most successful dieters we ever met once summed up her success by saying, "The best thing I ever did was buy a ton of fruit every week and keep it around all the time — even on my desk at work!"

3. FOR COOKING, CHOOSE MONOUNSATURATED FATS — namely, olive oil or canola oil (a popular brand of canola oil is Puritan); avoid highly saturated fats (butter and other animal fats, as well as coconut oil, palm and palm kernel oils, and cocoa butter — the fat in chocolate). We've taken care of the rest by designing our menus to limit your intake of polyunsaturated oils (safflower, corn, sunflower, soybean, etc.)

4. SWITCH FROM FRIED FOOD to baked, broiled, steamed or poached.

5. SWITCH FROM REFINED, LOW-FIBER CARBOHYDRATES (white flour, white bread, fruit juices) to high-fiber, complex carbohydrates. (By now, you know that we're talking about whole grains, fresh fruits, and vegetables).

6. REDUCE SALT INTAKE. Use "light" salt or a salt-free seasoning such as Mrs. Dash; buy low-sodium recipe ingredients, such as low-salt tomato sauce and tomato paste; and avoid high-salt products such as many canned soups; use fresh ingredients whenever possible, such as fresh mushrooms instead of canned.

7. EAT MORE FISH, especially cold saltwater varieties like tuna, salmon, herring, mackerel, pompano, shad, albacore, bluefish, sardines and halibut.

8. REDUCE YOUR STRESS LEVEL. Start by limiting daily caffeine consumption to two cups of coffee or strong tea, or four 12-ounce diet colas. And in Chapter Five, we'll explain how exercise helps to ease stress.

9. DRINK MORE LIQUID. Beyond the liquids taken with meals, you should be drinking extra water all day long, about eight 8-ounce glasses. Flavor with lemon juice or aspartame (artificial sweetener) if you like. You can also try mineral or seltzer water to provide the refreshing "bite" of carbonation (not soda or quinine waters, however, which are high in sodium).

Diet soft drinks are OK, as long as you follow the caffeine limit above and have no problem with artificial sweeteners. You may want to eliminate diet pop, however; research shows aspartame can stimulate appetites (more on that in a couple of pages).

10. EXERCISE. Yup, you've been meaning to start for ages. Maybe you were waiting until you could fit into that super-slim workout suit. C'mon, silly, start exercising now, so you *can* get into your dream wardrobe. (We'll get beginners started safely, and re-motivate those with exercise experience, in pages to come.)

A note on dairy products

Dairy products are the richest source for calcium, that crucial nutrient that science is finding helps prevent osteoporosis (or brittle bone disease). Osteoporosis strikes countless women after menopause.

A good supply of calcium also plays an important role in helping reduce high blood pressure and prevent colon cancer, according to recent studies by leading scientists, including two prominent researchers at Detroit's Wayne State University. [1]

But all too often, dairy products become partners with fat and/or sugar in the American diet. The best examples are whole milk and ice cream.

The vast majority of Americans, especially women, teenagers and low-income people (including many inner-city blacks and elderly persons) need less fat and fewer of sugar's empty calories in their diets. At the same time, most Americans need considerably more calcium than they get.

The Dee-troit Diet includes calcium from a variety of sources. Some readers may not be used to our Diet's frequent calls for yogurt, milk and other dairy products. We're careful to minimize added fat, however, by specifying non-fat yogurt, skim milk and other low-fat products. And while we schedule frequent servings of dairy products, each individual serving is modest. Studies have shown that small amounts of dairy products usually aren't a problem to the seven in 10 black Americans, and one in 10 whites, who have trouble digesting the lactose in dairy products — or to the many others who have varying degrees of other types of milk intolerance.

Research has shown that yogurt "with active cultures" (check the label; brands include Dannon, Yoplait and Columbo) has about 50 percent less of lactose, or milk sugar, making it much easier to digest than other dairy products for lactose-intolerant persons, who have trouble digesting most dairy products.

Says Ginnie Uhley of Dr. Lucas' clinics: "Usually, our lactose-intolerant patients — and many of them are blacks — aren't bothered by this diet at all. Most of them are bothered by the fat in dairy products. So the non-fat yogurt and the skim milk don't bother them nearly as much as whole milk, and they are keys to getting plenty of calcium."

This is a fairly calcium-rich diet, as well as a fiber-rich diet, but it doesn't have so much fiber that it will interfere with the calcium absorption, she says.

2

Basic
Rules
of the
Dee-troit
Diet: How
It Works

A little salty language

This diet averages 1,500 milligrams of sodium daily, which doctors consider a reasonable level. It's far below the 3,500 milligrams that Americans typically eat.

Still, those with hypertension (high blood pressure) may want to drop sodium intake even more, after checking with their doctors. They can do so by substituting low-salt seasonings in recipes calling for packaged seasoning mixes, such as the chili and ranch dressing mixes. They should also buy low-sodium recipe ingredients, such as low-sodium canned tomatoes and tomato paste.

At the table and in cooking, they can use salt-free products such as the Mrs. Dash line of seasonings. Keep in mind, the latest research shows that actual table salt (chemical name *sodium chloride*) has the greatest effect in raising blood pressure. Other sources of sodium, such as the flavor enhancer *monosodium glutamate*, seem to have less if any effect on blood pressure.

Yes, if you're like many people, the table salt you sprinkle on your food does raise your blood pressure.

Some straight talk on sugar

Sugar is not the diet demon we once thought it was. In a person with no weight problem, straight sugar by itself apparently causes little other permanent damage than potential tooth decay.

But sugar creates problems because of the company it keeps, and doesn't keep. Most sugar comes to us in combination with fats. Examples are chocolate, baked goods, ice cream, sugary glazes on meats and poultry skin, to name a few. And sugar's empty calories — with no accompanying vitamins, minerals or other nutrients — take up space in a diet that should be occupied by food you need to live your healthiest and perform your best.

Of course, in an overweight, under-exercised person, sugar contributes calories that, because they aren't burned off, become converted to body fat. Yuck! And sugar, especially when combined with fat, creates sensations of taste that often trigger overeating. You know, it really is easier to eat zero candy bars than to eat one.

While eschewing chocolate truffles, candy bars, cake and ice cream, the Dee-troit Diet does allow some sources of sugar. You can use low-sugar jams or jellies on bread and toast, bagels, rice cakes, even breakfast cereal and baked potatoes, if you like. A tablespoon or two certainly won't upset this diet and may make everyday foods more tasty for some dieters.

Also, the packaged dry seasoning mixes such as those in the chili and ranch dressing recipes tend to be fairly sweet.

Here are other ways to reward yourself with something sweet for sticking to Dee-troit Diet menus or faithfully doing our Dee-troit Plus workouts:

■ Sugar-free soda pop, including the Canfield's Diet Chocolate Fudge Soda that chocolate lovers swear by.

■ Sugar-free hot cocoa mixes, mixed with skim milk.

■ Knox Unflavored Gelatin, made into "Knox Blox" with fruit juice or an equivalent amount of sugar-free pop (see package directions), a refreshing, high-protein finger food that stores well in the refrigerator (and you can share with the kids, who'll love this).

■ Frozen fruit juice bars, made without added sugar (or buy popsicle

sticks and make your own in the ice cube tray).
■ Sherbets (some frozen yogurts are also low in fat; check labels for wording "made with skim milk" or "low-fat").

Check calorie counts on package labels to avoid over-rewarding yourself. Since all of the above are ultra-low in fat, none in moderation will upset the momentum of the Dee-troit Diet, say our nutritionists.

What about artificial sweeteners?

Aspartame, trade-named NutraSweet and Equal, is in diet pop and many other products. Most authorities, including government health experts, consider it safe. But here's something to consider.

If you're consuming a lot of aspartame, yet you're hungry all the time, take note of a study from England. It says aspartame may actually *stimulate* hunger pangs in some dieters about an hour after consumption.

Other research, by the American Cancer Society, shows that those using artificial sweeteners (typically saccharin) often have more trouble losing weight. Researchers think the reason is tied to the psychological freedom felt by users of sugar substitutes.

So use the sweet stuff sparingly, in whatever form. Of course, the best sweet snack is the natural sugar found in fruit.

For faster weight loss, purists may want to eliminate, as nearly as possible, all sources of sucrose. They can seek seasoning and chili mixes low in sugar, and use sugar-free substitutes to sweeten recipes.

No fruit juice allowed?

Here comes diet heresy, courtesy of the Lucas clinic. Fruit juice masquerades as a health food drink in the American way of eating. But to obesity experts, it's little better than soda pop.

Fruit juice contains lots of fruit sugar calories. And some — like cranberry and cherry — contain plenty of added refined sugar or corn syrup. More calories, in a package that doesn't fill you up and can be consumed in a flash.

Fruit juice drinkers miss out on the added vitamins in the pulp of fresh fruit, which also contains healthful fruit fiber, an aid to digestion that can help lower cholesterol. Fiber gives us a filled-up, satisfied feeling after a meal.

Adds Ginnie Uhley of the Lucas clinics: "You get sugar very rapidly when you drink juice, and anybody who needs to avoid getting sugar rapidly, including borderline diabetics and kids who tend to be hyper,

2

Basic
Rules
of the
Dee-troit
Diet: How
It Works

doesn't need that. We're talking about the equivalent of at least two tablespoons of sugar" in about four ounces of juice.

Instead of juice, the Dee-troit Diet offers several pieces of fresh fruit every day. For beverages, skim milk is in the diet. Otherwise, stick to coffee, tea, diet pop or water (limiting caffeine intake as in Rule No. 8 of the earlier section, Basic Rules of the Dee-troit Diet).

To lose, don't booze

Alcohol is a form of sugar. The limited benefit to cholesterol levels of moderate drinking has gotten plenty of media play. Once you achieve your target weight, a drink or two a day is acceptable, as long as your doctor agrees.

But during the weight-loss phase of Dee-troit Dieting, booze can bushwhack your best intentions. Here's why.

"Most alcoholic beverages are about 150 calories per serving, all sugar. Every extra 100 calories a day means 10 pounds a year in weight gain," assuming you do nothing to burn off the extra intake, says Dr. Lucas.

Furthermore, alcohol lowers inhibitions and whets appetites, so you're far less able to play it smart, diet-wise, after drinking. Booze sets anyone up for squandering a lot of great progress, and self-esteem, once weight loss is under way.

An exception is low-calorie cooking wine. In your own recipes, try using it to replace fats or oils. Although the alcohol in wine is high in calories, much of it evaporates during cooking, leaving the flavor of the wine behind.

Ease off on sugary snacks

By now, you know that two snacks per day are allowed on the Dee-troit Diet, as long as they're chosen from the approved list — and extra snacks are OK if you're tempted to cheat on the *wrong* foods.

But despite Americans' increasing tendency to skip balanced meals and snack all day, there are good reasons why you'll do better with three squares a day. The reason? Snacking will actually make you hungrier.

It seems the urge to snack can stem from a rebound effect in the brain and bloodstream resulting from earlier snacks!

Scientists say this is what happens: Between meals, as your body's energy levels fall, you may be tempted to reach for simple carbohydrates — candy or soda pop, for example. But after the resulting temporary rush of energy, sometimes accompanied by hyperactivity or anxiety, comes a release of insulin in the bloodstream, then a plunge in your blood sugar level. Translation? Your energy level droops. That, in turn, may trigger another carbohydrate craving — in other words, the urge for a "sugar fix". [2]

The alternative, when you crave something sweet? Aside from low-sugar jams and jellies, as mentioned above, your best bet is fruit.

Fruit is fairly low in calories, contains no fat, and its major sweet ingredient — fructose — is absorbed more slowly than other forms of ordinary sugar, or sucrose. That helps you avoid the rush-and-crash sugar cycle of snacking.

Fructose is also sweeter than sucrose, gram for gram. So less of it satisfies your sweet tooth. And eating fruit provides other nutrients such as Vitamin C and fiber, which clearly aren't present in your garden-variety glazed doughnut, candy bar or potato chip.

Remember, investing $5 or $15 in fruit, and always having a fresh bag in your car, near the TV, out in the kitchen, and next to your desk or workbench on the job, may be the cheapest weekly health insurance premium you ever pay.

2

Basic Rules of the Dee-troit Diet: How It Works

More water, please

One of the most successful dieters we know, a gourmet cook, diet recipe author and wife of a prominent physician in Scottsdale, Ariz., starts her day — and we're talking right after getting up! — by taking sips from a quart container of fresh, cool water.

By the time she leaves the house after breakfast, she's finished that quart.

The universal solvent is an important catalyst in aiding weight loss, says Dr. Lucas, for several reasons. First, "it's a substitute for food. Liquids distend your stomach and your bowel," fooling you into feeling full.

Second, water also flushes metabolized fats from the body after exercise, and helps prevent sagging skin during weight loss by keeping the skin plumped. [3]

Dieters should drink about two quarts of water a day — eight glasses of 8 ounces apiece. Some, but not all, can be coffee, tea or diet pop (see Rules No. 8 and 9 of the Basic Rules of the Dee-troit Diet).

Get the family involved

Don't go it alone. The Dee-troit Diet is designed so you can fix one meal for the whole crowd, delicious for everyone and legal for you.

If you're trying to lose weight and change bad eating habits into good ones, don't go it alone. Put the whole family on a low-fat, high-fiber diet like ours.

"Family participation is critical," says Dr. Lucas, to reinforce good habits. "This is a diet for the whole family, not just for weight loss but for maintaining current health or preventing future problems. You know, our kids' cholesterol levels are much higher than they should be. And a lot of our kids are just plain fat."

Not to worry — here comes help!

Do enjoy these weeks to come. Do feel better and look better. And do learn that quality food really can taste good.

Just read on for the next step in getting started.

---

[1] Michael Zemel, PhD, associate professor of nutrition and food science, and associate professor of endocrinology, Wayne State University; Gordon Luk, M.D., chief of gastroenterology, Harper Hospital in Detroit, and faculty member, Wayne State University School of Medicine.
[2] Bonnie Liebman, nutrition director, Center for Science in the Public Interest, Washington, D.C.
[3] Donald S. Robertson, M.D., MSc, founder of the Southwest Bariatric Nutrition Center, Scottsdale, Ariz., and co-author of "The Snowbird Diet" (Warner Books, 1986).

3

Winning the Numbers Game:
Don't Cut Calories,
Cut FAT Calories!

Up until now you've read lots about what you don't need, and some of what you do need, to lose weight while optimizing health.

Let's quickly learn a bit more about what your body craves for peak health and permanent weight loss. At the same time, we'll teach you some tricks for finding those good things in the maze of modern-day fat traps.

First, a few more diet reminders, to set up a vital principle

■ Don't use margarine. It's just as high in fat as butter!
■ You can blend non-fat chocolate extract, found in store baking sections, with skim milk and artificial sweetener to make chocolate milk.
■ Don't use non-dairy coffee "creamer," which is loaded with fat, often the most highly saturated kinds, such as coconut and palm oils.
■ Try substituting "soyburger" (soybean meat substitute) for hamburger or ground beef; another 'burger option is ground turkey, which is considerably lower in fat than beef.

And in place of ground meat in recipes like spaghetti sauce and chili, try omitting meat, or even substituting chopped vegetables. (We'll show you how in recipes that actually look and taste like they have bits of ground beef in them!)

■ Substitute matzo crackers or rice cakes for snack and soda crackers. It's amazing how much artery-clogging, diet-damaging fat is in the typical cracker.

■ Learn to enjoy the high-fiber goodness of a plain, unpeeled baked potato, one of the easiest snacks to make if you have a microwave oven. A plain baked potato has about 80 calories and is surprisingly high in Vitamin C. But adding a pat of butter adds about 35 calories of pure fat, while a tablespoon of sour cream kicks in 28. French-frying drives the count up far higher with *hundreds* of additional calories — all in belt-busting, cholesterol-laden fat.

■ Always check fat content on labels. Even though it's listed in grams, a mysterious volume of measure to most Americans, you can quickly learn the importance of relative amounts.

You'll find some surprises. For example, non-fat buttermilk is far lower in fat than whole milk; products labeled "low-salt" are sometimes very high in fat; and scads of frozen diet dinners are shockingly high in fat.

How can you make more sense out of those grams-of-fat listings on product labels, so that it's crystal clear EXACTLY how much fat you're getting? Read on.

A lesson in fat numbers

Now you're going to memorize a number and a fact, and learn what to do with them. It won't be hard, but it's more important than counting calories, even more important than checking your weight every morning.

It's a number that will help you suddenly make sense out of all the fine print and mysterious metric measurements on food product labels. The number is 9.

The fact you need to memorize is: There are 9 calories in a gram of fat. Got that? *One gram of fat has NINE calories.*

Knowing that, you can easily find out the number of fat calories in a serving of food. Just look on the product label for grams of fat, then multiply by 9.

For example, take milk. A cup of whole milk (eight ounces, that is) contains 8 grams of fat, as stated on the label. Now, 8 x 9 = 72. So, there are 72 calories of fat in that cup of milk.

So what, you ask? Wait, here's where the numbers get useful.

Just how much fat is that?
It's "moooo!" than you'd imagine

Let's find a way to put those 72 fat calories in perspective. We'll do it in this second part of this simple, but vitally important, math lesson.

If you're allergic to numbers, stay with us just another minute. You'll find that the next part is a key strategy for taking aim at fat calories everywhere, especially the hidden ones you may not even notice or enjoy. Yet those calories are making you overweight and unhealthy.

We're going to show you a simple formula for making extra sense out of the grams-of-fat listing on food labels. When we're done, we'll summarize the technique in a few lines, so you can cut it out if you need to, and post it or put it in your wallet, to help you remember the math when you need it.

(You'll find it's a cinch to compute with any pocket calculator. You can also do the figuring on paper; that's sometimes easier if you round off numbers to simplify. Occasionally, you'll find it's not hard to do this in your head. But most of the time, a calculator will make it lots easier).

Do you recall from your school days that part of something, divided by the whole of something, shows the percentage of that part to the whole?

Using math symbols, you can write Part ÷ Whole = Percentage of the Whole. The percentage can tell you if something has a smidgeon of fat in it, like 5 or 10 percent; or a fair amount, like 20 or 30 percent; or way too much, like 50 percent or even 99 percent!

To get the percentage of fat calories in a given food, you divide the part (that is, fat calories) by the whole (total calories). For that cup of milk, then, you would divide the number of fat calories (72) by the total calories in a cup of milk, which is also shown on the label (150).

The long division is 72 ÷ 150. Tossing that into your calculator, or working it out on paper for a minute, you'll find the answer is 48 percent. Wow, whole milk is 48 percent fat calories! That's more than double our Dee-troit Diet's 20 percent fat limit.

Let's compare that to so-called "2 percent" milk. That 2 percent is a misleading figure, as you shall see (it refers to the percentage of fat by weight, which is next to meaningless for nutritional insight).

Let's do the math together . . .
Grams of fat in one cup = 5 (from the label)
Total calories in a cup = 120 (from the label)
Now, 5 grams of fat x 9 calories per fat gram = 45 fat calories
Next, 45 fat calories ÷ 120 total calories = 37.5 percent

That means "2 percent" milk is actually about 38 percent fat calories! That's well over our Dee-troit Diet limit of 20 percent fat — although it's considerably less fatty than whole milk.

Sobering, isn't it, to learn that something labeled "2 percent milkfat" truly contains 38 percent fat calories, a figure that is 17 times greater?

This is why it's so important to get the calcium and protein from skim milk without the fat in other milks. Skim milk contains a mere trace of fat in eight ounces. So the percentage of fat calories is nearly zilch.

(Milk labeled "½ percent" contains 10 percent fat calories. That's within our diet limit, but to maximize your weight loss, use skim milk only.)

Now you know why it makes such a difference to calculate percentage of fat from product labels. We've summarized the formula below in a box that you can photocopy or clip out and paste to the back of your pocket calculator or front of your 'fridge . . . a simple reminder of some of life's most important numbers.

How to compute percentage of fat

(1 gram of fat = 9 fat calories)
_____ **(No. of fat grams) x 9 =** _____

To find percentage of fat, compute:
Fat calories ÷ total calories = percentage of fat
_____ **÷** _____ **=** _____ **% fat**

Now you know why it isn't enough, in fact it's downright misleading, to count calories. Dee-troit Dieters count the *calories that count*: fat calories.

Just a few seconds spent scanning labels and computing fat percentages can reveal some amazing differences among foods. For example, a 300-calorie slice of unfrosted white cake is about 33 percent fat — and worse if you add icing. But the same number of calories of angel food cake, a much more generous slice, contains almost *zero* fat calories (angel food cake is made without egg yolks or shortening). Believe it or not, a delectable slice of angel food cake covered with sliced strawberries is a *legal* Dee-troit Diet dessert. Watch for it!

Keep your eyes peeled!

From here on out, watch for grams of fat on everything you buy. Some products don't list it. You can avoid those or write the manufacturer to find out (and demand better labeling while you're at it!).

Knowing the fat formula above, you'll be able to evaluate, on the spot, just about everything you buy. Note the vital statistics on the following fat traps, listed in **bold print**, and note their low-fat substitutes, keeping in mind the Dee-troit Diet limit of 20 percent fat calories:

3

Winning the Numbers Game: Don't Cut Calories, Cut FAT Calories!

Fat content of common products

	Total Calories	Percentage of fat calories
Beans		
Canned beans with pork and sweet sauce (8 ounces)	383	**28%**
Canned red kidney beans (8 ounces)	230	4%
Heinz Vegetarian beans in tomato sauce (8 ounces)	230	4%
Fast food		
McDonald's Big Mac hamburger	570	**53%**
Kentucky Fried Chicken drumstick (original recipe)	147	**54%**
Roasted chicken breast without skin	284	19%
Burger King Whaler Fish Sandwich	488	**27%**
Plain baked potato (11 ounces)	290	almost 0%
Hardee's large french fries (113 grams)	381	**50%**
McDonald's Egg McMuffin	340	**42%**
Two large eggs, fried in butter	166	**65%**
Two soft-boiled egg whites (large eggs)	32	almost 0%
Egg Beaters egg substitute (¼ cup)	25	0%
Dairy products		
Whole milk (8 ounces)	150	**48%**
"2 percent" milk (8 ounces)	120	**38%**
"½-half percent" milk (8 ounces)	92	10%
Skim milk (8 ounces)	86	almost 0%
Whole-milk frozen yogurt (8 ounces)	260	**24%**
Plain non-fat yogurt (8 ounces)	110	almost 0%

Fat content of common products

	Total Calories	Percentage of fat calories
Salad dressings		
Mayonnaise (1 tablespoon)	100	**100%**
Hellmann's Light Mayonnaise (1 tablespoon)	50	**91%**
Weight Watchers Whipped salad dressing (1 tablespoon)	35	**67%**
Plain non-fat yogurt (1 tablespoon)	7	almost 0%
Kraft Reduced Calorie Buttermilk Dressing (1 tablespoon)	30	**90%**
Walden Farms Low Fat Ranch (1 tablespoon)	35	**51%**
Weight Watchers Italian Style (1 tablespoon)	6	almost 0%
Medford Farms No Oil Vinaigrette (1 tablespoon)	5	almost 0%
Kraft Oil-Free Italian (1 tablespoon)	4	almost 0%
Spreads		
Butter (1 tablespoon)	100	**100%**
Margarine (1 tablespoon)	100	**100%**
Fleischmann or Imperial diet (1 tablespoon)	50	**100%**
Peanut butter (1 tablespoon)	95	**76%**
Smucker's Apple Butter (2 teaspoons)	25	0%
Smucker's Low Sugar spreads (2 teaspoons)	16	0%
Featherweight Low Calorie Grape Jelly (1 tablespoon)	6	0%
Smucker's Imitation jams and jellies artificially sweetened (2 teaspoons)	4	0%
Pillsbury Artificial Vanilla Flavor Ready-to-Spread Frosting (serving)	160	**34%**
Baked goods		
Plain doughnut	180	**55%**
Raisin and honey bagel	200	5%
Pepperidge Farm Mint Milano cookies (3)	230	**51%**
Nabisco Chips Ahoy cookies (3)	140	**45%**
Nabisco 'Nilla Wafers (7)	130	**28%**
Gingersnaps (5)	147	18%
Nabisco Cherry or Blueberry Newton (3)	220	16%

Fat content of common products

	Total Calories	Percentage of fat calories
Fish		
Chunk Light Tuna in oil (2 ounces)	150	**78%**
Chunk Light Tuna in water (2 ounces)	60	15%
Van de Kamp's Microwave Light Breaded Cod (5-ounce fillet)	290	**59%**
Cod broiled with butter (5-ounce fillet)	243	26%
Cod broiled in white-wine sauce (5 ounces)	180	17%
Snack foods		
Potato Chips (½ ounce)	80	**56%**
Fritos Corn Chips (¾ ounce)	120	**53%**
Pretzels (1 ounce)	111	8%
Pillsbury Microwave Popcorn (2 cups, original flavor)	130	**52%**
Popcorn (2 cups air-popped, seasoned with Butter Buds liquid butter substitute)	46	almost 0%
Desserts		
Del Monte Tapioca Pudding (5 oz.)	180	20%
Weight Watchers Sandwich Bars (frozen, vanilla-flavor)	130	14%
Canfield's Chocolate Fudge Diet Soda (12 ounces)	2	0%
Pizza		
Fast-food pizza, cheese and pepperoni (two 12-inch slices)	380	**28%**
Fast-food cheese pizza (two 12-inch slices)	340	16%
Stouffer's Frozen Deluxe French Bread Pizza (6 ounces)	430	**44%**
Weight Watchers Deluxe Combination Pizza (7.25 ounces)	340	**32%**
Cereals		
Quaker 100 Percent Natural Cereal (¼ cup)	136	**40%**
Kellogg Cracklin' Oat Bran cereal (½ cup)	110	**33%**
Post Hearty Granola (1 ounce)	130	**28%**
General Mills Raisin Nut Bran cereal (½ cup)	110	**25%**
Kellogg Raisin Bran cereal (¾ cup)	120	8%
General Mills Wheaties (1 cup)	110	8%
Kellogg Mueslix Five Grain cereal (½ cup)	140	6%
Kellogg Product 19 (1 cup)	110	almost 0%
Post Natural Raisin Bran (½ cup)	80	almost 0%

3

Winning the Numbers Game: Don't Cut Calories, Cut FAT Calories!

Fat content of common products

	Total Calories	Percentage of fat calories
Candy		
Cadbury Almond candy bar (2 ounces)	310	**52%**
Snickers candy bar (56.7 grams)	274	**43%**
Necco Wafers (one roll, 57.3 grams)	160	0%
Nestle's Crunch (1.06 ounces)	160	**40%**
M&M, peanut (47.3 grams)	241	**45%**
Skittles (56 grams)	230	almost 0%

4

How to Spy Fat Traps
... in Food
and in Yourself

Hope we didn't bore you to tears with all those percentages in the last chapter.

The idea wasn't to have you wandering the supermarket aisles in a daze of long division. Instead, we wanted you to grasp this crucial idea of modern nutrition: that calorie counting is far less important than fat-calorie counting — and that some foods are drenched in fat while others have just a smidgeon.

By now we hope that you know the key to eating less fat. In fact, the key is limiting fat calories to no more than 20 percent of your diet.

By now, you've resolved to start checking food labels, counting grams of fat to cut your intake, once you begin Dee-troit Dieting.

Now, we're going to make life easy . . .

. . . on you AND your calculator! In this short section, we'll give you a shortcut for budgeting your fat grams, and finding out how many to allow each day. Here's how:

Again, start with your target weight. C'mon now, be realistic; this isn't a high school reunion. If your goal is 120 pounds, instead of multiplying by 10, this time *divide* by 10. That makes 12. Now, multiply by two. That's 24. Finally, add three. Total? It's 27, your daily limit of fat grams on the Dee-troit Diet. Now, pick up a pencil and figure your personal daily limit:

	You	Example
Your goal weight:	____	200
Divide it by 10:	____	20
Multiply it by 2:	____	40
Add 3:	____	43
And that's your very own daily limit of fat grams!		

Making the right choices

Now that you know your limit, keep count when you choose foods. You'll find some surprises, even among items you thought were sure diet bets. Consider these common examples:

■ **Tuna.** Before making a tuna sandwich for lunch, note the labels of water-packed tuna. In a two-ounce serving, Season brand has five grams of fat; Carnation two; Featherweight, a single gram. What a difference!

■ **Granola.** Now there's a word that rings diet chimes. Yet granola can be high in fat. Especially dangerous are granola bars. The fruit flavors of Quaker Chewy Granola Bars contain three fat grams. The chocolate chip and peanut butter versions have five. And the "Chunky Nut & Raisin" bar has six, making it 42 percent fat calories!

Other so-called "health" bars are higher. The apple-flavor Natural Nectar Fi-Bar, "fortified with oat bran" and coated with yogurt, is "a superior source of 12 dietary fibers," the label says. It also contains four grams of fat in 99 calories, giving it a calorie percentage of more than 36 percent fat.

■ **Muffins.** These tasty little cousins of cupcakes got a piping hot reputation when oat bran made health-food hitsville. Granted, oat bran muffins from low-fat recipes are legitimate means to reduce blood cholesterol. But many commercial muffins are so high in fat they defeat their purpose.

The package back of Heath Valley Fancy Fruit Muffins with Almonds

& Dates says, "Three muffins provide 50 grams of oat bran, 100 percent of the amount most often recommended each day to lower cholesterol." Yet each 170-calorie muffin contains six fat grams. Thus, three muffins contain 18 grams of fat — exactly two-thirds of the 27 fat grams allowed in a full day of the Dee-troit Diet's 1,200-calorie menu.

■ **Popcorn.** If you haven't heard, you must have been staring at the TV while munching: Microwave popcorn is loaded with fat! Forget the "Popcorn Plus Diet" book, forget those high-fiber wonders you've read about this fastest-growing snack food. A typical serving of microwave popcorn (2½ cups) has 11 grams of fat; butter-flavored ones have more.

If you insist on microwave brands, try Weight Watchers, with about one-sixth the fat of most others. Better yet, microwave or air-pop your own. You can douse the popcorn with Weight Watchers Buttery Spray, which has one fat gram per second of spray. But try popcorn without added fat, sprinkled with Mrs. Dash Salt-Free Seasoning. It's good!

■ **Frozen desserts.** When choosing a frozen dessert or fruit juice bar for snacks or dessert servings, check grams of fat. You'll find many Weight Watchers products that make diet sense, and some that don't. Weight Watchers Chocolate Mint, Vanilla and Double Fudge frozen bars each contain a single gram of fat. The Chocolate Mousse bar has even less. But the Chocolate Dip Ice Milk Bar has a surprising seven grams of fat.

Fruit juice bars that receive the Dee-troit Diet stamp of low-fat approval include the following: General Foods' Crystal Light Bars, Gold Mine Bullets Frozen Pops, Jell-O Gelatin Pops, Dole Fruit & Cream Bars, LifeSavers Flavor Pops, Melody Farms Twin Pops and Bomb Pop Jrs., Popsicle Ice Pops, Fudgsicle Ice Pops, Fudgsicle (brand) Fudge Pops (made with ice milk), and Welch's Fruit Juice bars.

Yogurt owns a comfy seat on the nutrition bandwagon, but only low-fat or non-fat yogurt holds a diet advantage. That rules out many frozen yogurts. Yoplait Soft Frozen Yogurt has three grams of fat in a miserly three-ounce serving. You're better off with Lite Lite Tofutti, a non-dairy product with less than one fat gram in four ounces.

At ice cream counters you can request nutrient counts for low-fat options. Most Baskin-Robbins (31 Flavors) shops offer "Low, Lite 'N Luscious." Two flavors contain two grams of fat, two other flavors have one gram, in four-ounce scoops. Just ask and you'll be handed a list showing the numbers. A same-size scoop of Baskin-Robbins' French Vanilla has a bathroom-scale-busting 18 grams of fat!

At Stroh and other ice cream counters, there are even better numbers. Both Skinny Dip Premium Low Calorie Frozen Dessert (in 10

4

How to Spy Fat Traps … in Food and in Yourself

flavors) and Columbo Soft Serve Lite Yogurt (five flavors) contain just a trace of fat per serving.

■ **Salad dressings.** Salad dressings, even those labeled "low-cal," are guilty until proven innocent.

Take the so-called "reduced calorie" versions of three dressings at Wendy's restaurants. Reduced Calorie Creamy Cucumber has five grams of fat per tablespoon. Reduced calorie Bacon/Tomato and Thousand Island dressings each contain a four-gram dollop of fat in every tablespoon. Since our plan strives for an average of 20 percent fat calories, and on a 1,200-calorie daily diet that imposes a limit of 27 fat grams daily, you'd blow off nearly a third of the day's 27 grams in one meal's salad dressing by using two tablespoons of those last two dressings.

In welcome contrast, Wendy's Reduced Calorie Italian dressing has only two grams of fat per tablespoon.

Supermarket dressings aren't safe, either, unless you take a second or two to scan fine print on the product backs. Don't rely on label fronts.

For example, Kraft Buttermilk Creamy Reduced Calorie Dressing has the words "less oil — fewer calories" crawling over its label front. But the label back says three fat grams per tablespoon.

When choosing a dressing, flip the bottle over and look for a listing that reads "0 grams fat" or "trace of fat" per tablespoon. On their fronts, these dressings will often say "no oil."

Some delicious examples are Kraft Oil-Free Italian, Medford Farms No-Oil Creamy Italian and Medford Farms No-Oil Vinaigrette, Wish-Bone Lite Italian and the Pritikin line of six dressings, including No-Oil Russian.

Just who do you think you are?

At this point, you know all the basic principles of Dee-troit Dieting and the rules to implement those principles. You know the numbers games and then some.

You could go out and start applying what you've learned right now. But besides missing out on the recipes and meal plans in this book, you'd be skipping an important part of our total formula for success.

What's that? Before we tell you, you need to talk to yourself a bit. Find out what kind of eater you are.

For starters, how's this for allaying guilt: Even if you're seriously overweight, the prime cause may not be overeating!

"There are well-known studies on this, but they haven't received a lot of play," says Dr. Lucas. The studies show that, fat or skinny, most people eat about the same number of calories. So what accounts for obesity?

It may be caused by eating the wrong food, especially products high in fat; or leading an inactive life; or inheriting the "biological or metabolic tendencies" to gain weight, says Lucas.

In many cases, however, overeating does play a part. Often, there's a combination of factors to blame, among them Americans' generally rich, high-fat diet and lives of relative leisure.

The antidote? We need to eliminate fat traps in our life-styles. Says Dr. Lucas: "What we have to do to treat overweight folks is to change their culture, take them out of their current habits, and give them a different kind of life-style — a different diet and a different activity level.

"So we take our theories and we say to the psychologist, 'OK, let's teach these people to exercise, let's teach these people to eat certain foods.' They do this by using psychological and behavior modification techniques. It's a retraining process. And in all that, we have to recognize that each person is different."

Find your eating personality type . . .

Dr. Lucas and his staff have observed a variety of personality types among their obesity patients. See if you recognize yourself:

1. EXPEDIENT EATER: This is a common obese personality in today's fast-paced society. Often workaholics, Expedients are obsessed with time management. They want instant food, and get plenty of fat in the bargain. They make fast-food runs, heat convenience food or dine from vending machines, promising to mend their ways once they've made that first million. If they ate the same number of calories in low-fat food, they probably wouldn't be overweight.

2. STRESS EATER: Also common. When under stress, Stressies reach for whatever food is handy to calm their nerves. Of course, they often have a favorite tranquilizer. It can be anything from gourmet chocolate to ordinary bread.

3. FOOD LOVER: This type just plain loves food, perhaps along with alcoholic beverages and other oral gratifiers. Food Lovers place no restrictions on themselves, and they may even cultivate social lives that revolve around wining and dining.

4. BORED EATER: This person is typically home a lot with little to do but eat. Low in energy, depressed, with few social outlets, Bored Eaters are

How to Spy Fat Traps ... in Food and in Yourself

4

the least likely type to exercise. But every time they pass the 'fridge, they do exercise one arm — reaching for calories.

5. BINGE EATER: Here, the problem is usually sweets, and in huge amounts. Some Binge Eaters alternate sweets with salty foods. Many are restrained most of the time. Then they lose control. Binge eating is tough to control and often requires professional counseling.

Find your non-exercising personality type . . .

Did you recognize yourself among the eating personalities? Now check your eating style against Dr. Lucas' personality types for activity. Note how many of the following groups correspond to various eating personality types.

1. TIME MIS-MANAGER: Many a Time Mis-Manager would like to exercise. Mis-managers know they should, but they're just too busy to cram workouts into busy schedules. The usual problem? Demanding careers, volunteer commitments and/or family lives (plenty are singles who are "married" to their jobs, adds Dr. Lucas). This activity type often corresponds with eating types 1 or 2, the Expedient Eater or the Stress Eater.

2. EX-JOCK OR EX-JOCKETTE: These hard-driving, high-achieving types can be workaholics, but they do take time for self-gratification. Once proud of their sporting bodies, they've channeled competitive urges into other pursuits, usually careers. Part of their inflated self-images includes lots of eating and drinking, and they have oversized waistlines to match. This type often corresponds to eating type 3, the Food Lover.

3. DISABLED EXERCISER: This type has a long-term disability, perhaps a back injury that never healed or a chronic illness. Exercise is an impossibility, or the Disabled thinks it is. Members of this group may be out of work, living on disability payments, perhaps even stuck at home for long periods. If so, a Disabled Exerciser easily become a Bored Eater (eating type 4).

4. INDOOR TYPE: This person loves sedentary activities. Indoor types have time to exercise but absolutely no interest. They prefer to pursue relaxing pastimes from crochet to chess, photography to poker, shop work to stamp collecting, books to the boob tube. Some also love cooking and eating, and they become Food Lovers (as in eating type 3). Others have a secret activity to accompany their other hobbies: compulsive eating. And still others simply lead such inactive lives that weight gain is inevitable.

What to do . . . .

. . . if you fit one or more of these personality types? Truly irrational behavior such as binge eating calls for counseling, and perhaps drug treatment. And if you have a major obesity problem (50 or more excess pounds) you should get professional help.

But most people need only a push in the right direction to improve their diets and their health. Says Dr. Lucas: "People who don't have a major problem, all they need is a little bit of fine-tuning in one or two areas and they'll do much better."

1. KEEP A DIARY. Before you start the Dee-troit Diet, try writing down every single thing you put in your mouth for three days, and jot down a word or two about the time of day and circumstances. You'll soon learn where problems lie.

For example, perhaps you're an Expedient Eater, wolfing dinners while standing up in the kitchen, grabbing anything in reach. You'll need to change, to plan meals and sit down to eat slowly for more satisfaction and balanced nutrition. And you'll end up being more efficient at your work because you'll be stoking your furnace with higher quality food.

Nope, smart low-fat eating doesn't have to take up your day — check out our convenience meals in the chapters to come. It's even possible in fast-food restaurants!

2. PLAN A NON-FOOD LIFE-STYLE. Don't center your social life around pizza parlors and fast-food restaurant runs. Schedule activities that don't involve food, and cultivate friends who have non-eating interests. One good interest to share is exercise. Find walking partners by posting your name on bulletin boards where you work, go to school or worship.

3. GET OUT OF THE HOUSE. Again, exercising may be a great way to get yourself away from the 'fridge. Take long walks and re-discover everything about your neighborhood. Find a friend to join you for more fun and positive reinforcement.

4. JOIN A GROUP. Overeaters Anonymous groups around the country offer a very low-cost means of social support, even crisis lines that provide instant, friendly volunteer counseling virtually any time of day or night. There are no weigh-ins, dues or fees. Check your local telephone listings for the Overeaters Anonymous group nearest you. Here's the address of the national Headquarters: P.O. Box 92870, Los Angeles, Calif. 90009.

4

How to Spy Fat Traps ... in Food and in Yourself

Another national group that helps members control eating is TOPS — for Take Off Pounds Sensibly. Hundreds of thousands of members can't be wrong. Here's the address of TOPS' national headquarters: 4575 S. Fifth Ave., Milwaukee, Wis. 53207.

5. READ THE NEXT CHAPTER. It's that very important part of our total Dee-troit Diet formula for success that we've just hinted at so far. By now, you know what we're talking about.

5

Anyone's Exercise Plan:
It Really Does Burn Off Fat

There's nothing that can make losing weight more painless than exercise.

Without changing a thing about the food you choose or how much you eat, exercise can turn the calorie expenditure tables in your favor.

The idea is simple: If you eat the same as usual while burning up more calories than you're consuming, you start losing weight. And if you change to a low-fat diet at the same time you begin exercising, your progress can be significant.

Best of all, exercising tones up lean body tissue, the good-looking pounds we *don't* want to shed; at the same time, exercise zeroes in on fat cells, to burn them as fuel. All the while, exercise helps by letting you eat enough calories for optimum health and vitality while still losing weight.

In contrast, crash dieters, on ultra-low-calorie diets, run the risk of losing attractive lean body tissue during weight loss, leaving them with sagging, unattractive skin and flesh that continues to have more fat cells than needed. At the same time, they don't get enough food for good nutrition, a further risk to vitality and appearance.

Finally, in case after case, exercising gives dieters a psychological edge, an extra boost of motivation and self-confidence that helps cement the change to healthier eating and slimmer living — for good.

"We know that even a little bit of exercise seems to help, because in weight-loss programs those who exercise do much better," says Dr. Lucas.

"It may be that it just ties together your whole commitment to weight loss. A runner will say, 'Hey, I'm not about to go out and ruin all this training by eating badly.' ... If I'm exercising to improve my cholesterol level, I'm not going to eat eggs afterward."

You're too busy to exercise?

Who isn't? You're probably saying, "Wow, this book is doling out more than my already jammed schedule can handle!"

Wait. Before you skip this exercise chapter, please consider:

■ The time you may spend, sooner or later, seeking treatment for illness if you don't lose weight and get fit.

■ The increased self-esteem and efficiency you'll miss out on (perhaps even job promotions and romance) if you skip the opportunity to look and feel your best.

■ The ways that moderate exercise and healthful living habits can become part of everyday activities, so that you hardly know you're burning calories or living a healthier life.

■ The pleasant, stress-fighting surprise you can expect. Countless exercisers find that, whether it's a half-hour walk or 90 minutes of rough-and-tumble racquetball, exercise can be a wonderfully positive way to relieve stress and free-floating anxiety. Instead of taking a mental and physical toll on health — as do alcohol, tranquilizers, excessive sleep or TV watching — exercise leaves you refreshed and ready for more efficient work or more enjoyable play.

Consider these points and you may discover you're too busy NOT to exercise!

First, a few cautions

If you've been inactive for some time, check with your doctor. The American Heart Association suggests that before starting a vigorous exercise program, you should get a checkup if you're over 35, if there's a history of heart disease in your family, if you're a smoker or former smoker, or if you have a history of diabetes or other medical problems.

See a sports medicine specialist if you suffer from chronic back pain, shin pain or have foot problems that might interfere with exercising (however, remember that excess weight or a sedentary life-style can be the cause of just such medical ailments).

Now, let's get started

The Dee-troit Diet exercise plan has three components. Doing all three is best; two is OK; at the very least you should do one.

Here they are: 1. Aerobic workouts (such as walking and cycling); 2. Non-aerobic workouts (stretching and toning); 3. Workaday workouts (like taking the stairs at work instead of the elevator, to wean yourself just a little from our all-American dependence on labor-saving devices).

All three will help you speed your weight loss and become a fitter person. Here they are, in order of importance.

1. AEROBIC EXERCISE: This is the kind of exercise that can light your personal fat-burning fire. It's any activity that provides brisk, continuous exertion, raising the heartbeat and breathing rate. For most beginners, walking or stationary cycling are best.

Those who are already at a modest level of fitness can jog, swim, cross-country ski, do aerobic dance or other vigorous sports. But walkers and stationary cyclists will get comparable benefits with less risk of injury. In addition, walkers need no special equipment beyond comfortable shoes with cushioned soles.

Says Dr. Lucas: "Start by walking a very short distance. It could be as little as a quarter of a mile (perhaps to the end of your block and back) at a very slow, comfortable pace. Very gradually, increase the distance.

"This ought to be done five days a week. Seven days is a little too much," because it can lead to injuries, he says.

Two or three days a week is OK at first, says Dr. Lucas. But your ultimate goal should be to exercise aerobically for 45 minutes, five days a week.

Sound like a lot? Many obesity clinic patients put in a full hour, five days a week. And they're still leading far less physical lives than their ancestors of just a generation or two ago.

Take the diabetic woman in her late 50s who came to Dr. Lucas' clinic with a laundry list of serious health problems, including high cholesterol on top of her diabetes symptoms. Today, those problems are gone or well under control. So are 66 pounds, thanks to low-fat dieting and her hour-long stints — five times weekly — on an exercise cycle. She no longer needs insulin. The bonus? She can justify watching all her favorite TV shows while she cycles!

2. NON-AEROBIC EXERCISE: We've just said that aerobic exercise is what burns fat and makes every body system flash a green light for health.

But there are days that people can devote no more than five or 10

5

Anyone's Exercise Plan: It Really Does Burn Off Fat

minutes to exercising. That's when non-aerobic exercise can help, by limbering and toning stiff, flabby muscles, and helping release nervous and muscle tension, which can trigger false hunger pangs.

While stretching and toning are no substitute for a brisk half-hour or 45-minute walk when it comes to weight loss, they can help round out the Dee-troit Diet exercise plan by alleviating sources of chronic back pain and relaxing muscles tightened in previous bouts of aerobic activity.

Simple stretches take only seconds a day but can relieve tension and backache, while keeping you relaxed and comfortable during fat-burning exercising. Don't tug on muscles to limber up; a gentle, prolonged pull as you exhale is safer!

3. WORKADAY WORKOUTS: Someday you're going to join that expensive health club, right?

But meanwhile, you can't possibly take the stairs at work when the elevator is beckoning. And you can't possibly park a block from the store you're headed for. Or could you?

Remember, every calorie you expend in your daily routine can be that much more weight down the drain. Recent research shows that some people burn as many as 800 calories a day just by fidgeting.

While we aren't going to give you lessons at tapping your feet or drumming your fingers, we do want to slip more physical activity into your daily life. We'll tell you a new way to do that each day in a later chapter.

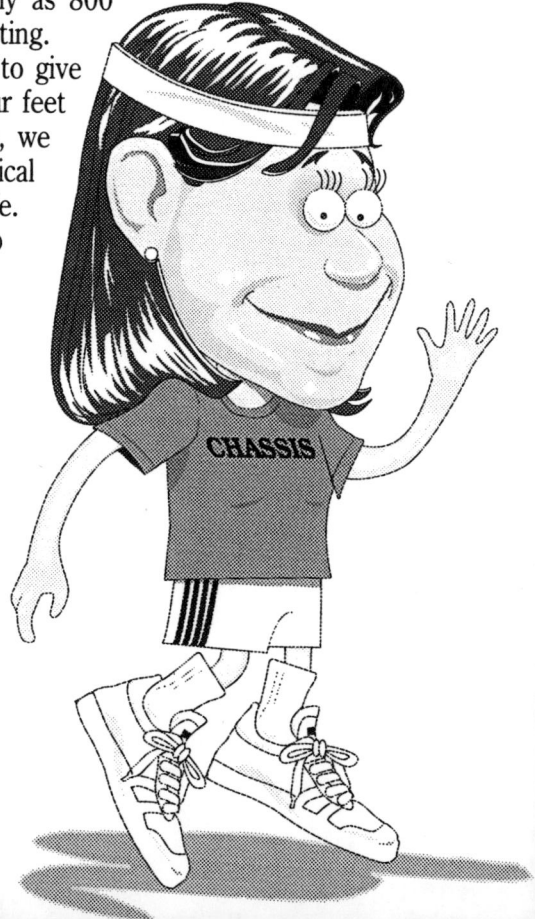

Walk your way to health and weight loss

If you've never done any exercise before, or not in years, start by walking for just 10 minutes. Don't feel you have to rush. Your pace is much less important than finishing the full 10 minutes without stopping.

In your first week of Dee-troit Dieting, work your way up to 15 minutes of non-stop walking, in each of five workouts that week. After that, just add five minutes to your workouts every other week.

Here's the schedule, based on research with hundreds of overweight patients at Dr. Lucas' obesity clinic:

Walking schedule, five days a week

Week 1 .... 10-15 minutes	Weeks 7-8 .... 30 minutes
Week 2 .... 15 minutes	Weeks 9-10 .... 35 minutes
Weeks 3-4 .... 20 minutes	Weeks 11-12 ..... 40 minutes
Weeks 5-6 .... 25 minutes	Weeks 13-14 ..... 45 minutes

Your goal is clear: Be able to walk briskly or do other vigorous exercise for 45 uninterrupted minutes after a 12-week build-up.

Here's how to pace yourself. After the 12 weeks, you should be walking at least two miles in those 45 minutes. Beyond 12 weeks, you can stay with a 45-minute workout, but pick up the pace so the distance you walk (or run, swim or cycle) increases by 10 percent a week.

Two or three days a week is OK at the very beginning (although more often will speed your weight loss), but the sooner the better that you reach five days of exercise a week, with two rest days dispersed throughout the week.

Eventually you'll be striding three miles in 45 minutes, five times a week. And you'll be in great shape!

By the way, Dr. Lucas takes plenty of his own medicine. He's finished more than a dozen marathons since he started running a decade ago. For years, he's used the latest research findings to help others slim down. But his own health credo, he says, is eight centuries old — simply put by a Hebrew physician named Maimonides who just might have been the ideal Dee-troit Dieter:

"Eat lightly and run to breathlessness."

5

*Anyone's
Exercise
Plan: It
Really
Does Burn
Off Fat*

Burn it, baby, burn it

Check this list to see how you can burn off 1,000 calories a week, at the same time you tone muscles and relieve stress:

Calories used by various activities

Activity	Calories per hour
Aerobic dancing	500
Basketball	400
Bowling	150
Cross-country skiing	1,000
Dancing (slow)	125
Dancing (fast)	350
Downhill skiing (½ day)	400
Jogging	720

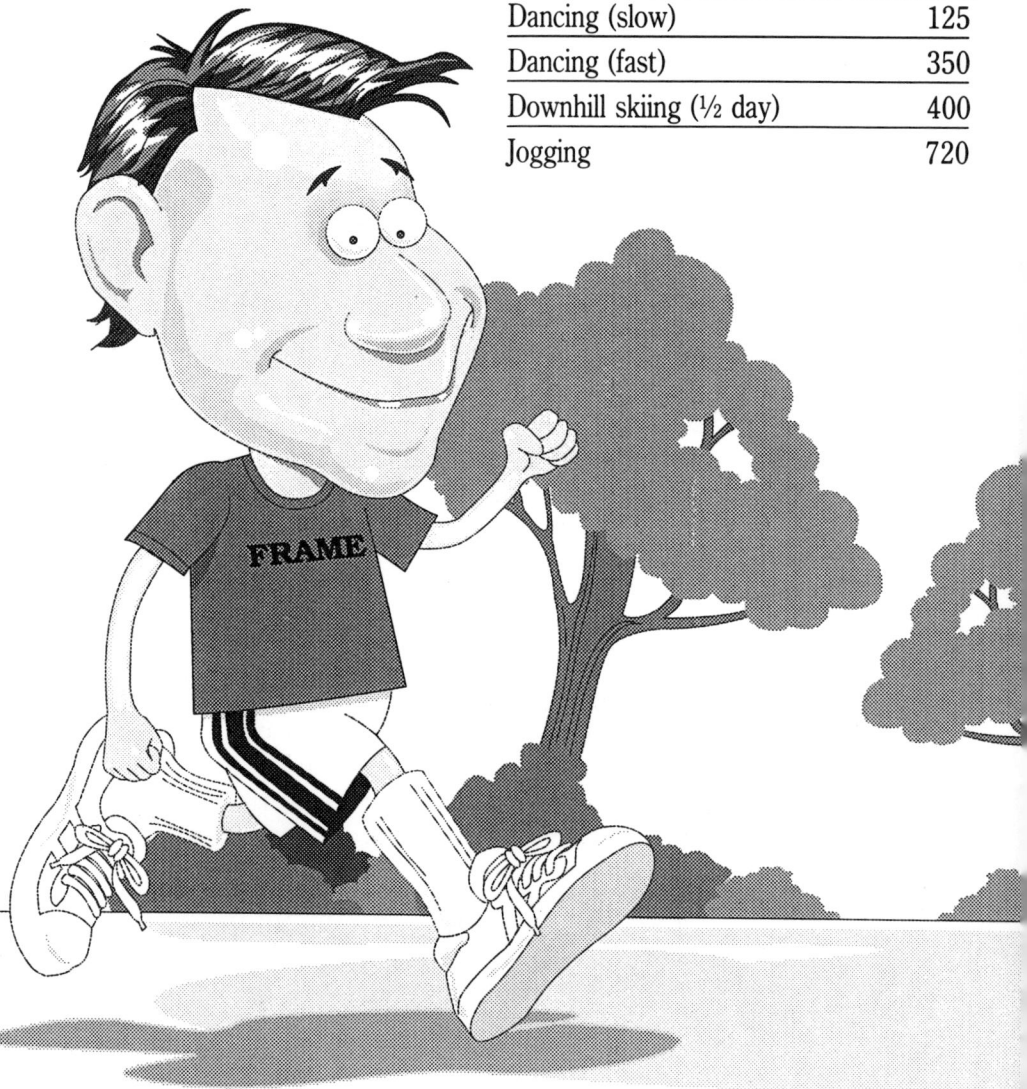

Activity	Calories per hour
Racquetball	350-550
Rowing machine (vigorous)	750
Stair climbing	1,050
Stationary cycling (moderate)	450
Swimming (moderate)	500
Table tennis	175
Walking (easy pace)	250

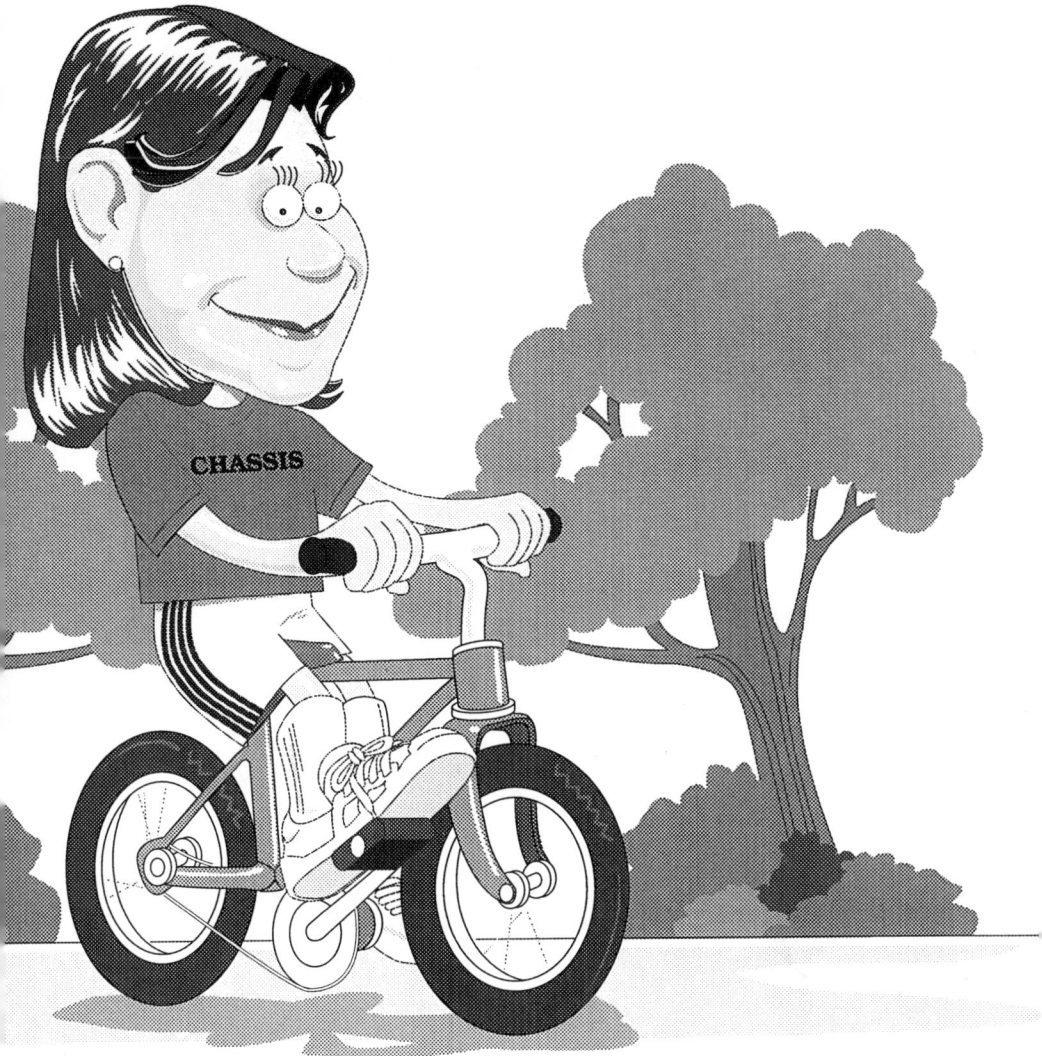

Source: President's Council on Physical Fitness, Washington, D.C.

You really CAN do it

The experience of hundreds of obesity patients says you can.

After you make exercise a habit, and see how much better it makes you look and feel, you'll find it gets easier and more fun. The challenge lies in overcoming Sir Isaac Newton's famous law of inertia: A body at rest tends to stay at rest.

Once you get started, you'll see the truth in the second part of Newton's law: A body in motion tends to stay in motion.

Still, let's be frank. We know it isn't easy to change a life of, ahem, *sloth.* You're going to have to make your body sweat a bit, get up earlier, stretch things that don't want to stretch at first, and say *no thanks* to things you're accustomed to.

You'll have to think, too, in the coming weeks — about what you're eating in restaurants, what you're cooking at home, what time to go to bed, even how you spend your lunch hour.

But we're going to make it as easy as we can. Good tasting, too! Now, go to the next chapter to get started on the Dee-troit Diet!

6

Week I of the Dee-troit Diet

Here's a quick preview of the diet weeks to come:

WEEK I: CONVENIENCE WEEK. Super-fast recipes combined with restaurant meals and frozen dinners.

WEEK II: CONVENIENCE CONTINUED. More of the above.

WEEK III: FAMILY DINNER WEEK. Seven days of simple lunches combined with recipes the whole family will enjoy; a special exercise schedule, too.

WEEK IV: COMBINED WEEK. A combined selection of of family dinners and convenience/restaurant choices; hints on how to lower your cholesterol level at mealtimes, too.

Y ou can start Dee-troit Dieting anytime, but our menu plans are designed around a Sunday-through-Saturday weekly cycle. We suggest you read through a week of menus on Sunday, make your choices, then do your shopping and some cooking for the week that same day. Thus, Day 1 would be a Sunday, Day 2 would be a Monday, Day 6 a Friday (whoa, pizza day!), and so on.

Our menus are strategically designed to balance important nutrients through the week. We aim for variety and you should, too. Still, if you want to trade any breakfast, lunch or dinner for another breakfast, lunch or dinner, feel free to do that.

Before jumping into the first menu, check off these reminders to help our plan work for you all week:

■ **Get your fiber:** Whenever possible, include high-fiber, whole-grain food in every meal. Examples are whole wheat bread (but not "cracked" wheat or bread that's dark simply because of added molasses or food coloring); whole wheat rolls, pasta and bagels, too; and brown rice, which takes only a few minutes longer to cook than white. Purchase oat bran and wheat (or "miller's") bran, and add them to cereals, pancakes, meat loaf, whatever you cook at home (some people carry a couple tablespoons of bran in a plastic bag for adding to restaurant food). Oat bran helps lower blood cholesterol; wheat bran is an excellent source of bulk for aiding digestion. Bran is available at health food and bulk food stores and an increasing number of supermarkets.

■ **Eat fruit:** You should eat fruit where indicated on meal plans and also as snacks. Two 80-calorie snacks are allowed each day on our 1,200-calorie plan, and fresh fruit makes a great, filling, sweet snack. To obtain another type of fiber that improves blood cholesterol levels, include grapefruit or oranges every week.

■ **Dodge the salt:** Look for low-salt and no-salt versions of supermarket foods and condiments. Avoid adding salt to foods. Use no-salt condiments such as herbs or Mrs. Dash salt-free seasonings. In restaurants, you can ask that little or no salt be used in food preparation.

■ **Drink lots of liquid.** Eight large (8-ounce) glasses of water or other liquid per day is a Dee-troit Diet must.

Week I of the Dee-troit Diet

We'll start you out on the Dee-troit Diet with a week that mixes at-home recipes and brown-bag lunches with frozen dinner choices and even several fast-food selections.

At the same time, we'll accelerate your early fat loss by setting daily nutrient totals slightly below our general 20 percent fat limit on calorie intake.

As if you didn't know: Restaurant and processed foods tend to be high in fat, cholesterol and sodium; and low in fiber and other nutrients. To fight back, we've singled out the most nutritious selections around. Now, enjoy . . . And whatever you do, don't let yourself get hungry! (Eat extra approved snacks if necessary, because they won't add fat, just fill you up.)

GROCERY LIST

Before buying, scan the full week's menus and choose your preferences. Some meals offer several options among at-home recipes and restaurant meals.)

Breakfasts

■ Eggs (whites only) or Egg Beaters (egg substitute);
■ Raisin bran (such as Post Natural Raisin Bran) or other unsweetened breakfast cereal;
■ Skim milk;
■ Whole wheat bread;
■ Low-sugar jam or jelly;
■ Fresh fruit, including bananas, to have with or on cereal;
■ Low-fat vanilla yogurt (no more than 200 calories per cup);
■ Oat bran (available in health and bulk food stores and in some supermarkets, often as Mother's Oat Bran Creamy High-Fiber Hot Cereal or Sovex Oat Bran Hot Cereal).

Everyday use

Depending on which daily meals you choose, you'll need varying amounts of:
■ Vegetarian vegetable or tomato soup, your choice;
■ Bread (whole wheat for daily use; rye for Day 5 lunch);
■ Low-sugar jam or jelly;
■ Orange or lemon sherbet;
■ Skim milk;
■ Plain non-fat yogurt; selection of low-sugar fruit-flavored yogurt (such as Dannon "25 percent less sugar" yogurt);
■ Frozen fish or chicken dinners (no more than 320 calories and 7 grams fat per serving);
■ Frozen fruit juice bars (limit of 90 calories and 1 gram fat);
■ Lettuce;
■ Green peppers;
■ Cooking onions and green onions;
■ Tomatoes.

6

Week I of the Dee-troit Diet

■ Optional: bean sprouts; plenty of fresh fruit, including citrus fruits; Pam cooking spray; olive, canola or safflower oil for cooking; powdered butter substitutes such as Butter Buds or Molly McButter; "no-oil" salad dressings (look for "0 grams fat" per serving); fresh or frozen mixed vegetables; frozen juice bars such as Dole or Shamitoff.

Recipe ingredients

DAY 1 Turkey Dinner: For serving six and having leftovers for sandwiches, buy a 7-pound turkey breast, or buy a full bird and freeze leftovers.

"Make sure you don't buy a self-basting bird. These have been injected with oils. Use fresh or frozen turkey, and cook it on a rack so it doesn't absorb fat as it cooks," advises Tom Violante, owner of the Holiday Market in Royal Oak, Mich.

DAY 2 Tossed Salad (and following days): at least 2 heads of lettuce, 2 green peppers, 1 large bunch of green onions, 1 package of carrots, 1 package of celery. Optional: tomatoes and bean sprouts.

DAY 2 Creamy Low-fat Dressing (and following days): lemon juice, ¾ cup low-fat cottage cheese (1 percent milk fat); small onion; garlic clove; dill and pepper.

DAY 2 Frozen Dinner: Choose a microwave-type or other frozen fish or chicken dinner with no more than 7 grams of fat and 320 calories per serving; check labels carefully, avoiding those with cream sauces or breading.

DAY 3 At-home Dinner Choice (alternative is Wendy's restaurant dinner): large potato, 16-ounce can Heinz Vegetarian Beans (optional: chili powder and green onion).

DAY 4 Lunch: 6½-ounce can of water-packed tuna, one 24-ounce container of low-fat cottage cheese (1-percent milk fat), stalk of celery, whole wheat bread or pita bread.

DAY 4 Turkey Rice Casserole Dinner: Rice, pound of ground turkey, 1 medium cooking onion, 4 medium carrots, fresh mushrooms, small zucchini, 6-ounce can Spicy V-8 Juice or tomato juice; egg white.

DAY 5 California Melt Lunch: Rye bread, zucchini, fresh mushrooms, carrots, green pepper, ½-cup shredded mozzarella cheese, large sweet onion.

DAY 6 At-home Lunch (alternative is Taco Bell lunch): Non-cream meatless vegetable or 2 small cans or 1 large can of tomato soup (preferably low-salt; check label: no more than 2 grams fat per serving); whole wheat bread; low-sugar jam or jelly; orange or lemon sherbet.

DAY 7 Lunch: Same soup as Day 6 or cup of low-fat, low-sugar fruit-flavored yogurt (such as Dannon "25 percent less sugar" types); 2 slices whole wheat bread or plain bagel; carrot and celery.

DAY 7 Hurry Tuna Curry Dinner: Rice, onion, green pepper, 8-ounce can of plain non-fat yogurt, 8 ounces of Land O Lakes Lean Cream or similar sour cream substitute, curry powder, 6½-ounce can water-packed tuna.

6

*Week I
of the
Dee-troit
Diet*

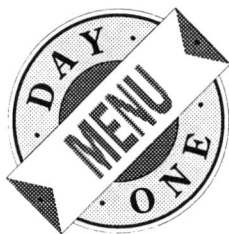

These are approximate nutritional totals for Day 1, not including two approved 80-calorie snacks: about 1,230 calories, 59 grams protein, 11 grams fat, 224 grams carbohydrate, 1,055 milligrams sodium, 219 milligrams cholesterol, 8 percent fat.

Breakfast

Three-quarters cup of Post Natural Raisin Bran or serving of other unsweetened dry cereal (maximum of 120 calories and 1 gram of fat per serving; check labels). Slice 1 banana over cereal. Fresh citrus fruit (whole orange or half-grapefruit), eaten separately. Cup of skim milk. Black coffee, tea or ice water. Total: about 330 calories, 4 grams protein, 1 gram fat, 76 grams carbohydrate, 307 mg sodium, 4 mg cholesterol, 3 percent fat.

Lunch

Serving of Legal Scrambled Eggs (recipe follows). Two slices of bread, toasted, preferably whole wheat; spread with 2 tablespoons low-sugar jam or jelly. Piece of whole, fresh fruit. Total: about 367 calories, 14 grams protein, 8 grams fat, 61 grams carbohydrate, 401 mg sodium, 120 mg cholesterol, 20 percent fat.

Dinner

Four ounces of fresh roasted skinless turkey breast (recipe follows). One-half cup of any fresh or frozen green vegetable or mixed vegetables (without sauce), steamed or microwaved, topped with ½ teaspoon Butter Buds Sprinkles (butter-flavored seasoning), or lemon juice, and pepper if desired. Medium baked potato, served with ½ teaspoon Butter Buds sprinkles (or teaspoon of liquefied Butter Buds powdered mix) or Molly McButter Sprinkles (All-Butter flavor, or Sour Cream and Butter flavor). Fast Waldorf Salad (recipe follows). Total: about 532 calories, 43 grams protein, 2 grams fat, 87 grams carbohydrate, 347 mg sodium, 95 mg cholesterol, 3 percent fat.

Reminders

■ Coffee, tea or diet pop are optional with all meals, but limit caffeine to two cups coffee or strong tea, or four 12-ounce cola beverages, per day (you may want to eliminate diet pop, however; research shows aspartame can stimulate appetites).

■ Two 80-calorie snacks are allowed per day (See Chapter Two for the 80-Calorie Snack List).

Use extra snacks or adjust meal portion sizes to achieve a daily calorie count that's right for your target weight (see Chapter Two). But if you find you're hungry, eat more of the legal snacks. Dee-troit Dieters should never feel nagged by hunger pangs.

■ Don't forget to exercise (see Chapter Five).

6

Week I of the Dee-troit Diet

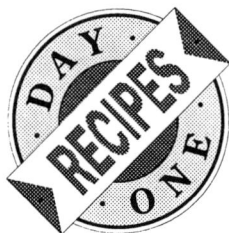

Roast Turkey

For serving six and having leftovers for sandwiches, use a 7-pound turkey breast. Or you can buy a full-sized bird and freeze leftovers.

Pre-heat oven to 450 degrees. Spray turkey skin lightly with Pam cooking spray. Put turkey breast in baking pan with skin side up (cavity down). Insert meat thermometer in turkey flesh so it is not touching bone or the pan. Put turkey in oven, reduce heat to 375. Cook until meat thermometer says 170 degrees (10 to 20 minutes per pound; check thermometer often). Remove from oven. Allow to cool 10 to 15 minutes. Remove skin and discard. Slice turkey meat and serve.

(Note: You can bake potatoes at the same time, putting them in the oven for about 20 minutes, after piercing skin with a fork.)

Nutrition details per 4-ounce serving: about 154 calories, 34 grams protein, 1 gram fat, 0 grams carbohydrate, 59 mg sodium, 95 mg cholesterol, 6 percent fat.

Legal Scrambled Eggs

½ teaspoon vegetable oil (preferably canola, olive or safflower), plus oil for skillet surface
½ cup chopped onion
½ cup chopped fresh mushrooms (about 4 large or a 4-ounce can)
½ cup chopped green pepper
3 whites of medium eggs
1 egg yolk
   Splash of skim milk (about 2 tablespoons)
   Pepper and Mrs. Dash Salt-Free Seasoning to taste

Using a paper towel moistened with vegetable oil, wipe inside surfaces of a non-stick skillet. Then place half teaspoon of oil and chopped onion in the skillet over medium high heat. Saute several minutes. Add mushrooms and green pepper; saute an additional 2-3 minutes. Place egg whites and yolk in a bowl. Whisk for 10 seconds with splash of skim milk, then pour into skillet and scramble. Season to taste with pepper and salt-free seasoning.

Serves two.

■ **Nutrition details per serving:** about 114 calories, 7 grams protein, 6 grams fat, 8 grams carbohydrate, 81 mg sodium, 120 mg cholesterol, 48 percent fat.

Fast Waldorf Salad

4   tablespoons raisins or dried currants
4   stalks celery, diced
4   medium apples, cored and diced
8   tablespoons low-fat vanilla yogurt
    Optional: lemon juice (after dicing apples, you can sprinkle lightly with lemon juice to keep flesh from turning brown)

Toss ingredients in a large bowl.
Makes six servings.

■ **Nutrition details per serving:** about 96 calories, 1 gram protein, trace of fat, 23 grams carbohydrate, 37 mg sodium, 2 mg cholesterol, about 3 percent fat.

■ **Note:** For a less sweet, tangier salad, omit vanilla yogurt and use 4 tablespoons plain non-fat yogurt mixed with 4 tablespoons Weight Watchers Reduced Calorie Salad Dressing (mayonnaise-type).

6

*Week I
of the
Dee-troit
Diet*

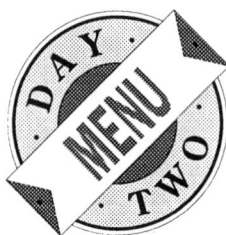

These are approximate nutritional totals for Day Two with Breakfast A and averaging lunch choices (not including two 80-calorie snacks): about 1,200 calories, 65 grams protein, 12 grams fat, 208 grams carbohydrate, 2,200 mg sodium, 59 mg cholesterol, 9 percent fat.

Breakfast

Choose A or B.

A. Two egg whites, or equivalent serving of egg substitute such as Egg Beaters (soft- or hard-boil whole eggs, removing yolks after cooking). One slice of whole wheat toast spread with up to 1 tablespoon low-sugar jam or jelly (can substitute one-half cup of unsugared raisin bran, such as Post Natural Raisin Bran). Cup of skim milk or plain non-fat yogurt. One-half grapefruit or other whole fresh fruit. Total: about 250 calories, 16 grams protein, 1 gram fat, 48 grams carbohydrate, 380 mg sodium, 4 mg cholesterol, 4 percent fat.

B. Breakfast shake: ½ large banana, 1 cup low-fat vanilla yogurt, ¼ cup skim milk, 2 tablespoons oat bran. Mix ingredients in blender on high until blended. Total: about 288 calories, 15 grams protein, 3 grams fat, 47 grams carbohydrate, 181 mg sodium, 12 mg cholesterol, 9 percent fat. (Tip: Even if you don't like yogurt try this; *everybody* loves it.)

Lunch

■ **Restaurant suggestions:** Elias Bros. Big Boy "Health Smart" lunches.

A. Vegetable Stir Fry. Serving of rice. Skim milk (10 ounces). Vitari strawberry dessert. Total: about 494 calories, 19 grams protein, 6 grams fat, 92 grams carbohydrate, 1,278 mg sodium, 7 mg cholesterol, 12 percent fat.

B. Cabbage soup (bowl). Two slices whole wheat bread (with preserves). Skim milk (10 ounces). Sliced banana plate. Vitari strawberry dessert. Total: about 488 calories, 20 grams protein, 1 gram fat, 100 grams carbohydrates, 1,052 mg sodium, 14 mg cholesterol.

■ **Do-it-yourself lunch:** 12-ounce bowl of non-cream meatless vegetable or tomato soup (preferably low-salt type; check label: no more than 2 grams of fat per serving). Two slices of bread (preferably whole wheat) with 2 tablespoons low-sugar jam or jelly. Whole piece of fruit or sliced fruit plate without dressing. Scoop of orange or lemon sherbet (quarter cup, 70-calorie serving). Cup of skim milk. Total: about 500 calories, 18 grams protein, 6 grams fat, 94 grams carbohydrates, 1,718 mg sodium, 4 mg cholesterol, 11 percent fat.

Dinner

Frozen dinner. Choose a microwave-type or other frozen fish or chicken dinner with no more than 7 grams of fat and 320 calories per serving; check labels carefully, avoiding those with cream sauces or breading. Small Tossed Salad with 2-3 tablespoons of store-bought no-oil dressing or Creamy Low-Cal Dressing (salad and dressing recipes follow). Frozen fruit juice bar.

We chose Stouffer's Lean Cuisine Chicken A L'Orange with Almond Rice. Total: about 548 calories, 41 grams protein, 7 grams fat, 81 grams carbohydrate, 636 mg sodium, 51 mg cholesterol.

Reminders

■ Coffee, tea or diet pop are optional with all meals, but limit caffeine intake to two cups of coffee or strong tea, or four 12-ounce cola beverages, per day.
■ You're allowed two 80-calorie snacks per day; see Chapter Two for list.
■ Juice bar limit: 90 calories, 1 gram fat.
■ Don't forget to exercise.

6

*Week I
of the
Dee-troit
Diet*

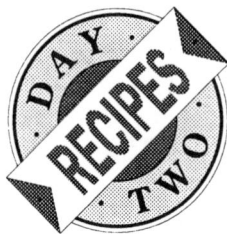

Small Tossed Salad

⅓ medium head lettuce, shredded
⅓ green pepper, sliced
⅓ cup chopped green onion, carrot and celery,
     mixed to taste
2 slices tomato (optional)
¼ cup bean sprouts (optional)

Toss together lettuce, green pepper, onion, carrot, celery, and tomato if desired. Top with bean sprouts if desired.
Serves one.
■ **Nutrition details per serving:** about 40 calories, 2 grams protein, 0 grams fat, 8 grams carbohydrate, 35 mg sodium, 0 mg cholesterol (for tomato and sprouts, add 15 calories).

Creamy Low-Cal Dressing

¼ cup skim milk
1 tablespoon lemon juice
¾ cup low-fat cottage cheese (1-percent milk
     fat)
½ small onion
1 clove garlic, crushed
½ teaspoon dill weed
     Pepper to taste

Combine ingredients in a blender. Blend on high for 1 minute. Makes 1 cup.
■ **Nutrition details per tablespoon:** about 11 calories, 1 gram protein, less than 1 gram fat, 1 gram carbohydrate, 37 mg sodium, 1 mg cholesterol, 8 percent fat.

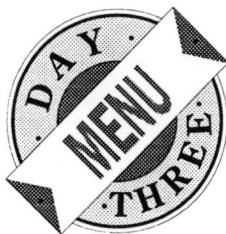

These are approximate nutritional totals for Day 3, with Breakfast A, Dinner B and averaging lunches (not including two 80-calorie snacks): about 1,100 calories, 71 grams protein, 17 grams fat, 168 grams carbohydrate, 2,150 milligrams sodium, 119 milligrams cholesterol, 14 percent fat.

Breakfast

Choose A or B from Day 2, or choose any breakfast from the Substitute Breakfast page in the Appendix.

Lunch

A. Country Turkey sandwich: 2-ounce slice of roasted skinless turkey (use leftover turkey from Day 1) or skinless chicken; serve between two slices of whole wheat bread or inside 1 round of pita bread (6-inch diameter), spread with 2 tablespoons plain non-fat yogurt; serve with with lettuce leaves and one-half sliced tomato. Cup of skim milk. Whole fresh fruit. Optional: slice of onion for sandwich. Total: about 380 calories, 30 grams protein, 5 grams fat, 53 grams carbohydrate, 500 mg sodium, 50 mg cholesterol, 12 percent fat.

B. McDonald's Chicken Salad Oriental with 2-ounce packet of Oriental or Lite Vinaigrette dressing and packet of Chow Mein Noodles. Orange juice (6 ounces). Total: about 362 calories, 26 grams protein, 6 grams fat, 52 grams carbohydrate, 1,010 mg sodium, 80 mg cholesterol, 15 percent fat.

Dinner

A. Wendy's Potato with Chili. Order plain baked potato (specify "no butter on it!") and a serving of chili (9 ounces). Glass of ice water. Spoon chili over potato; do not eat soda crackers included with chili. Total: about 480 calories, 27 grams protein, 11 grams fat, 68 grams

6

Week I of the Dee-troit Diet

carbohydrate, 1,020 mg sodium, 50 mg cholesterol, 21 percent fat. (Be sure to have a fresh fruit snack and cup of skim milk before or after dinner.)

B. At home: Large baked potato, served with 8-ounce can of Heinz Vegetarian Beans poured over potato (heat beans first; if desired, stir in ⅛ teaspoon chili powder, 1 chopped green onion, and pepper to taste). Small Tossed Salad with 2 tablespoons Creamy Low-Fat Dressing or store-bought "no-oil dressing). (see Day 2 recipes; store-bought dressing must list "0 grams fat" on label). Whole piece of fruit. Frozen fruit juice bar. Total: about 535 calories, 19 grams protein, 3 grams fat, 106 grams carbohydrate, 1,630 mg sodium, no cholesterol.

Reminders

■ Coffee, tea or diet pop are optional with all meals, but limit caffeine intake to two cups of coffee or strong tea, or four 12-ounce cola beverages per day.

■ Juice bar limit: 90 calories, 1 gram fat.

■ You're allowed two 80-calorie snacks per day; see Chapter Two for list.

■ Don't forget to exercise.

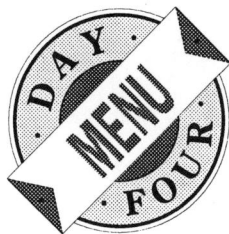

These are approximate nutritional totals for Day 4 with Breakfast A, not including two 80-calorie snacks: about 1,230 calories, 86 grams protein, 13 grams fat, 196 grams carbohydrate, 1,930 mg sodium, 120 mg cholesterol, 10 percent fat.

Breakfast

Choose A or B from Day 2, or choose any breakfast from the Substitute Breakfast page in the Appendix.

Lunch

Tuna sandwich: Mix 3½ ounces (half a small can) of drained water-packed tuna (preferably low-salt type) with 2 tablespoons of low-fat cottage cheese (1-percent milkfat only!) and 1 tablespoon of chopped celery (optional: add 1 tablespoon chopped green onion). Serve between 2 slices of whole wheat bread; or add several lettuce leaves and stuff inside the halves of 1 round of pita bread (6-inch diameter). Whole fresh fruit. Cup of skim milk. Total: about 436 calories, 43 grams protein, 3 grams fat, 59 grams carbohydrate, 550 mg sodium, 69 mg cholesterol, 6 percent fat.

Dinner

Turkey Rice Casserole (recipe follows). Cup of skim milk. Small Tossed Salad (see Day 2 recipes) with 2 tablespoons "no-oil" dressing (label must say 0 grams fat). Frozen fruit juice bar. Total: about 544 calories, 27 grams protein, 9 grams fat, 89 grams carbohydrate, 1,000 mg sodium, 47 mg cholesterol, 15 percent fat.

Reminders

■ Coffee, tea or diet pop are optional with all meals, but limit caffeine intake to two cups of coffee or strong tea, or four 12-ounce cola

6

*Week I
of the
Dee-troit
Diet*

beverages, per day.
■ You're allowed two 80-calorie snacks per day; see Chapter Two for list.
■ Juice bar limit: 90 calories, 1 gram fat.
■ Don't forget to exercise.

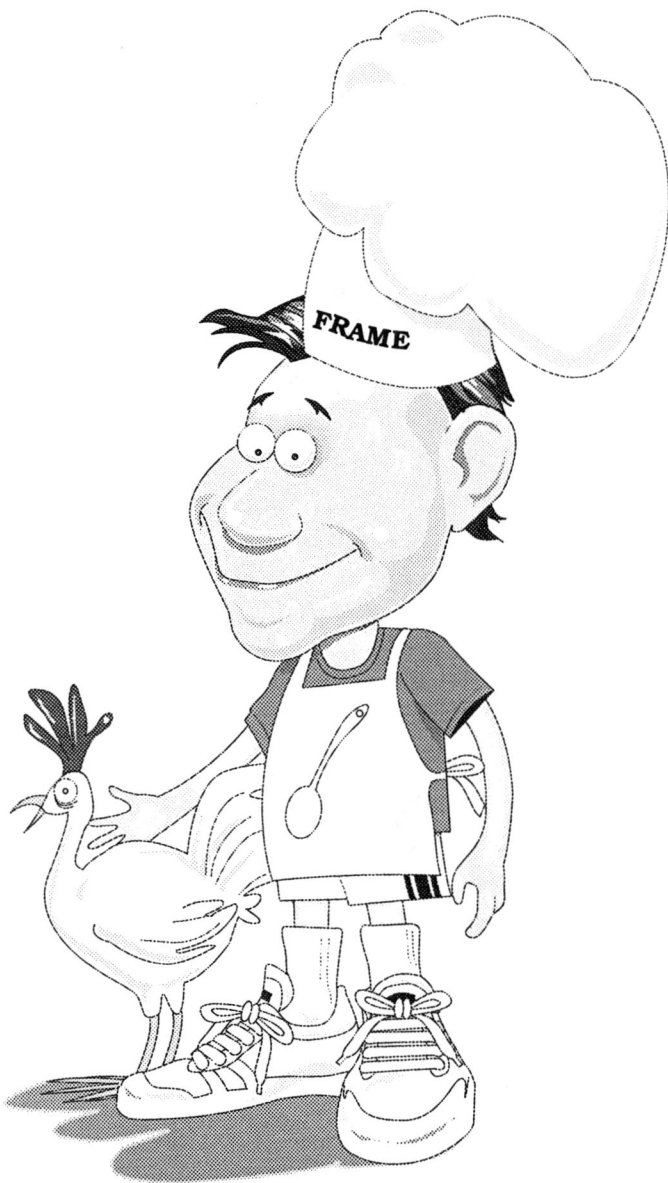

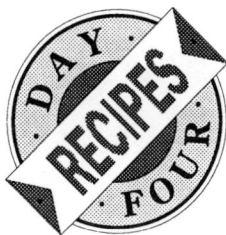

Turkey Rice Casserole

1½ cups rice (uncooked)
1 pound ground turkey (fat and calories are
    even lower if you chop turkey leftovers from
    Day 1 recipe instead of buying commercially
    ground turkey)
1 cup chopped onion
4 medium carrots, diced or sliced into small
    pieces (about 1 cup)
4 large mushrooms, diced (about 1 cup)
½ small zucchini, diced (about ¾ cup)
1 6-ounce can of Spicy V-8 juice (or tomato
    juice with teaspoon of pepper mixed in)
1 egg white

Preheat oven to 375 degrees. Begin cooking rice according to
package directions. In large bowl, combine turkey, onion, carrots,
mushrooms, zucchini, juice and egg white; mix by kneading with clean
hands. After rice has cooked 10 minutes or more, drain and reserve
liquid. Cool rice by rinsing and re-draining, then mix rice evenly into
turkey mixture. Press into casserole dish that has been sprayed with
cooking spray such as Pam (or wiped with vegetable oil and paper
towel). Pour reserved rice liquid over casserole dish. Bake covered at
375 for 30 minutes; remove cover and bake additional 15 minutes.
    Serves six.
■ **Nutrition details per serving:** about 316 calories, 16 grams
protein, 8 grams fat, 47 grams carbohydrate, 192 mg sodium, 43 mg
cholesterol.

6

*Week I
of the
Dee-troit
Diet*

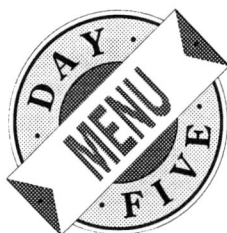

These are approximate nutritional totals for Day 5, with Breakfast B, California Melt lunch, and frozen fish dinner (not including two 80-calorie snacks): about 1,120 calories, 71 grams protein, 16 grams fat, 170 grams carbohydrate, 2,850 milligrams sodium, 78 milligrams cholesterol, 13 percent fat.

Breakfast

Choose A or B from Day 2, or choose any breakfast from the Substitute Breakfast page in the Appendix.

Lunch

A. California Melt open-face sandwich (recipe follows). Cup of skim milk. Whole fresh fruit. Cup of non-cream meatless vegetable or tomato soup (preferably low-salt type; check label: no more than 2 grams of fat per 8-ounce serving). Total: about 347 calories, 18 grams protein, 5 grams fat, 56 grams carbohydrate, 1,230 mg sodium, 12 mg cholesterol.

B. Cup of low-fat, low-sugar fruit-flavored yogurt (such as Dannon "25 percent less sugar" types). Two pieces of whole wheat bread or 1 plain bagel (spread with 2 tablespoons low-fat jam or jelly). One-half carrot and 1 celery stalk, sliced into strips. Total: about 400 calories, 14 grams protein, 6 grams fat, 74 grams carbohydrate, 360 mg sodium, 14 mg cholesterol, 14 percent fat.

Dinner

Restaurant suggestions: Elias Bros. Big Boy "Health Smart" dinners:

A. Cajun Cod or Broiled Cod with rice or potato; bowl of sliced bananas or strawberries; Vitari frozen desert. Total: about 553 calories, 55 grams protein, 9 grams fat, 60 grams carbohydrate, 800 mg sodium,

89 mg cholesterol, 11 percent fat.

B. Cajun Chicken with potato or rice; bowl of strawberries or sliced bananas. Vitari frozen dessert. Glass of skim milk (10 ounces). Total: about 618 calories, 53 grams protein, 9 grams fat, 81 grams carbohydrate, 583 mg sodium, 74 mg cholesterol, 10 percent fat.

At home: Frozen dinner. Choose a microwave-type or other frozen fish or chicken dinner with no more than 7 grams of fat per serving; check labels carefully, avoiding those with cream sauces or breading. We chose Weight Watchers Fillet of Fish Au Gratin with Broccoli, about 220 calories, 24 grams protein, 6 grams fat, 17 grams carbohydrate, 660 mg sodium, 50 mg cholesterol. Serve with 1 slice whole wheat bread or toast. Small Tossed Salad (see Day 2 recipe) with 2 tablespoons "no-oil" dressing (must list "0 grams fat" on label). Cup of skim milk. Frozen fruit juice bar. Total: about 518 calories, 38 grams protein, 8 grams fat, 71 grams carbohydrate, 1,540 mg sodium, 54 mg cholesterol, 14 percent fat.

Reminders

■ Coffee, tea or diet pop are optional with all meals, but limit caffeine intake to two cups of coffee or strong tea, or four 12-ounce cola beverages, per day.

■ You're allowed two 80-calorie snacks per day; see Chapter Two for list.

■ Don't forget to exercise.

6

*Week I
of the
Dee-troit
Diet*

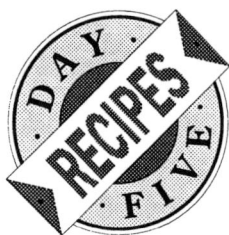

California Melt

4   slices rye bread, toasted
¾   cup shredded zucchini or alfalfa sprouts
1   cup sliced fresh mushrooms
½   cup shredded carrot
2   tablespoons chopped green pepper
½   cup shredded mozzarella cheese
¼   cup large sweet onion rings (uncooked)
    Dash of seasoning salt (optional)

Arrange toasted bread on microwave-safe serving plate. Top each with zucchini or sprouts, mushrooms, carrot, green pepper, cheese and onion rings. Sprinkle with seasoning salt if desired. Microwave on full power (rotating once) for 1½-2 minutes or until cheese melts; or oven-broil 3 minutes until cheese melts.

Makes 4 open-faced sandwiches.

■ **Nutrition details per serving** (1 sandwich): about 114 calories, 7 grams protein, 3 grams fat, 17 grams carbohydrate, 285 mg sodium, 8 mg cholesterol, 21 percent fat.

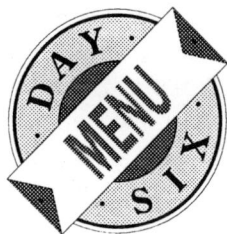

These are approximate nutritional totals for Day 6, with Breakfast A, Lunch A and Pizza Dinner, but not including two 80-calorie snacks: about 1,140 calories, 51 grams protein, 28 grams fat, 175 grams carbohydrate, 1,900 mg sodium, 38 mg cholesterol, 22 percent fat.

Breakfast

Choose A or B from Day 2, or choose any breakfast from the Substitute Breakfast page in the Appendix.

Lunch

A. Taco Bell: Bean Burrito and iced tea or coffee. Total: about 360 calories, 12 grams protein, 11 grams fat, 54 grams carbohydrates, 850 mg sodium, 14 mg cholesterol, 28 percent fat. (Be sure to have 1 whole fresh fruit as a snack before or after meal).

B. Do-it-yourself lunch: 12-ounce bowl of non-cream meatless vegetable or tomato soup (preferably low-salt type; check label: no more than 2 grams of fat per serving). Two slices of bread (preferably whole wheat) with 2 tablespoons low-sugar jam or jelly; whole piece of fruit or sliced fruit plate without dressing. Scoop of orange or lemon sherbet (quarter cup, 70-calorie serving). Cup of skim milk. Total: about 500 calories, 18 grams protein, 6 grams fat, 94 grams carbohydrates, 1,718 mg sodium, 4 mg cholesterol, 11 percent fat.

Dinner

Pizza night: Order meatless cheese pizza "with half the cheese"; optional: green pepper, onion and mushroom toppings.

Example: Little Caesars Pizza take-out meal. Three slices medium Cheese Pizza with Individual Tossed Salad and 1½-ounce packet of Little Caesars Low-Calorie Italian Dressing. With diet pop, ice water or artificially sweetened iced tea. Total: about 528 calories, 23 grams

6

*Week I
of the
Dee-troit
Diet*

protein, 16 grams fat, 73 grams carbohydrate, 1,473 mg sodium, 20 mg cholesterol, 27 percent fat. Optional: onion, green pepper and mushroom pizza toppings (add 40 calories).

Or: Pizza Hut restaurant meal. Two slices of a medium or three slices of small pizza, "Thin 'n Crispy" style only (*not* "Personal Pan Pizza"). Large tossed salad of lettuce and vegetables (salad bars include broccoli, cauliflower, beets, tomato, cucumber, mushrooms, onion and garbanzo beans; do *not* use bacon bits, cheese or egg slices, or any Pizza Hut salad dressing; dress salad with squeezes of lemon wedge, available on request or comes with iced tea). With diet pop, ice water or artificially sweetened iced tea. Total: about 430 calories, 28 grams protein, 14 grams fat, 48 grams carbohydrate, 900 mg sodium, 33 mg cholesterol, 29 percent fat. Optional: onion, green pepper and mushroom pizza toppings (add about 40 calories).

Reminders

■ Coffee, tea or diet pop are optional with all meals, but limit caffeine intake to two cups of coffee or strong tea, or four 12-ounce cola beverages, per day.

■ You're allowed two 80-calorie snacks per day; see Chapter Two for list.

■ Don't forget to exercise.

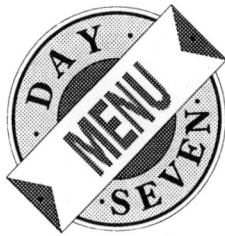

These are approximate nutritional totals for Day 7, using Breakfast B and Lunch B, and not including two 80-calorie snacks: about 1,200 calories, 55 grams protein, 15 grams fat, 209 grams carbohydrate, 941 mg sodium, 43 mg cholesterol, 11 percent fat.

Breakfast

Choose A or B from Day 2, or choose any breakfast from the Substitute Breakfast page in the Appendix.

Lunch

A. Soup lunch: 12-ounce bowl of non-cream meatless vegetable or tomato soup (preferably low-salt type; check label: no more than 2 grams of fat per serving). Two slices of bread (preferably whole wheat) with 2 tablespoons low-sugar jam or jelly. Whole piece of fruit or sliced fruit plate without dressing. Scoop of orange or lemon sherbet (quarter cup, 70-calorie serving). Cup of skim milk. Total: about 500 calories, 18 grams protein, 6 grams fat, 94 grams carbohydrates, 1,718 mg sodium, 4 mg cholesterol, 11 percent fat.

B. Yogurt lunch: Cup of low-fat, low-sugar fruit-flavored yogurt (such as Dannon "25 percent less sugar" types). Two pieces of whole wheat bread or 1 plain bagel (spread with 2 tablespoons low-fat jam or jelly). One-half carrot and 1 celery stalk, sliced into strips. Total: about 400 calories, 14 grams protein, 6 grams fat, 74 grams carbohydrate, 360 mg sodium, 14 mg cholesterol, 14 percent fat.

Dinner

Serving of Hurry Tuna Curry (recipe follows), poured over 1 cup cooked rice. One-half cup of any fresh or frozen green vegetable or mixed vegetables (without sauce), steamed or microwaved, topped with ½ teaspoon Butter Buds Sprinkles (butter-flavored seasoning), or lemon juice, and pepper if desired. Cup of skim milk. Total: about 514 calories, 26 grams protein, 6 gram fat, 88 mg carbohydrate, 400 mg sodium, 54 mg cholesterol, 10 percent fat.

6

Week I of the Dee-troit Diet

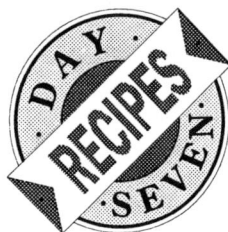

Hurry Tuna Curry

4 cups rice (cooked)
½ cup chopped onion
1 cup chopped green pepper
1 8-ounce container plain non-fat yogurt, at
   room temperature
8 ounces Land O Lakes Lean Cream or equivalent low-fat sour cream substitute, at room
   temperature
   Curry powder and pepper to taste
1 6½-ounce can of water-packed tuna, drained

Cook rice according to package directions. When done, remove from heat and leave covered to keep hot.

Spray inside of large non-stick skillet with cooking spray such as Pam. Place onion and green pepper in skillet; cook over medium heat for several minutes until onions are clear and peppers are slightly softened. Reduce heat to low. In a bowl, mix yogurt and Lean Cream. Stir in up to 1 tablespoon curry powder, to taste, and up to ¼ teaspoon pepper, to taste. Add yogurt/sour cream mixture to skillet, stirring. Add tuna, stirring continuously for 1-2 minutes until thoroughly mixed and warmed through. Do not overcook. Divide rice evenly among 4 plates. Spoon mixture over plates of rice.

Serves four.

■ **Nutrition details per serving (without rice):** about 140 calories, 10 grams protein, 5 grams fat, 15 grams carbohydrate, 200 mg sodium, 54 mg cholesterol, 29 percent fat.

7

Week II
of the Dee-troit Diet

Here's another week of convenience dieting — recipes you can fix quickly along with more restaurant meals and frozen dinners that meet our diet guidelines.

First, a few tips about ordering in restaurants. Salad bars are the proverbial diet trap. They can be low-calorie, nutritious and filling — or just the opposite if you dump ladles of high-fat dressing on rabbit food.

Even restaurant dressings labeled "low-cal" may be shockingly high in fat. Avoid creamy and cheesy types, like "low-cal" Thousand Island, blue cheese and creamy Italian. Reduced-calorie French and Italian seem best. Even so, spoon them on in limited amounts — no more than a couple of tablespoons. (Note: Low-calorie Italian may use aliases like "light vinaigrette" or "low-cal oil and vinegar.")

To be sure, bring your own dressing in your purse or pocket. Buy single-serving packets of "no-oil dressings" at the supermarket (brands include Estee and Featherweight).

Here are other salad bar fat traps to avoid:

■ Pre-mixed salads: Restaurant versions (like cole slaw or bean, pasta or potato salads) tend to be be high in fat.

■ Bacon bits, crumbled boiled egg yolks and cheese: All are high in saturated fat and cholesterol.

■ Seeds, chow mein noodles, olives and croutons: Small tidbits, but shockingly high in fat.

Now for the good stuff: Load up on fresh goodies, including carrots, sprouts, cabbage, tomato slices and fruit slices.

Pickles are acceptable, although a bit high in sodium. Garbanzo beans also rate an OK. While slightly fatty, they compensate by containing soluble fiber, same as peas and kidney beans, helping improve cholesterol levels. They also contain a modest amount of protein. Sliced boiled egg whites are also a good source of low-fat protein.

GROCERY LIST

Breakfasts

You'll need eggs (whites only) or Egg Beaters (egg substitute); raisin bran (such as Post Natural Raisin Bran) or other unsweetened breakfast cereal; skim milk; whole wheat bread; low-sugar jam or jelly; fresh fruit, including bananas, to have with or on cereal; low-fat vanilla yogurt (no more than 200 calories per cup); oat bran (available in health and bulk food stores and in some supermarkets, often as Mother's Oat Bran Creamy High-Fiber Hot Cereal or Sovex Oat Bran Hot Cereal).

Everyday use

Whole wheat bread and bagels; skim milk; selection of fresh fruit (grapefruit, oranges, bananas, apples); frozen fruit juice bars (Shamitoff, Dole, Borden or other brand; juice bar limits are 90 calories, 1 gram fat); lemons or reconstituted lemon juice; no-oil salad dressings; non-stick cooking spray; low-sugar jam or jelly.

Lunches

DAY 1 Sandwich: Can of water-packed tuna, low-fat cottage cheese (1-percent milkfat), celery stalk.

DAYS 2-5: restaurant or at-home meals using everyday ingredients.

DAY 6 Soup: 10-ounce package of frozen asparagus or broccoli; chicken-flavored bouillon cubes (preferably low-salt); minced onion flakes or onion salt; ½ cup evaporated skim milk; fresh or dried parsley.

Also, fixings for a tossed salad (lettuce and your choice of cucumber, carrot, tomato, bean sprouts, other vegetables).

Dinners

DAY 1 Clam Pasta Dinner: 6½-ounce can of clams; 2 cloves of garlic, 3 green onions, cornstarch, dry white wine (optional), parsley (fresh or dried), 8 ounces (uncooked) spinach fettuccine or other pasta (ordinary spaghetti is fine). Frozen peas or other vegetable.

DAY 2 Frozen Chicken Dinner: Choose a microwave-type or other frozen chicken dinner with no more than 7 grams of fat and 320 calories per serving; check labels carefully, avoiding those with cream sauces or breading.

DAYS 3-5: restaurant dinners.

DAY 6 Frozen Fish Dinner: Same fat and calorie rules as Day 2.

DAY 7 Vegetarian Burritos Dinner: 16-ounce can of Heinz Vegetarian Beans; plain non-fat yogurt; low-sodium V-8 juice; tomatoes, green peppers and onions; lettuce; pita bread, 6-7 inches in diameter; Mrs. Dash Extra-Spicy Salt-Free Seasoning.

7

*Week II
of the
Dee-troit
Diet*

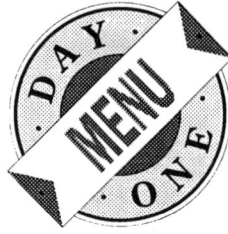

Here are today's approximate nutritional totals, using Breakfast A and not including two 80-calorie snacks: 1,200 calories, 85 grams protein, 11 grams fat, 195 grams carbohydrate, 1,120 mg sodium, 135 mg cholesterol, 8 percent fat.

Breakfast

Choose A or B.

A. Two eggs whites (or equivalent serving of egg substitute such as Egg Beaters). Prepare soft- or hard-boiled (remove yolks after cooking). One slice of whole wheat toast spread with 1 tablespoon low-sugar jam or jelly (can substitute ½ cup of unsugared dry cereal, such as Post Natural Raisin Bran; maximum of 120 calories and 1 gram of fat per serving; check labels). Cup of skim milk. One-half grapefruit or other whole fresh fruit. Black coffee, tea or ice water. Total: about 250 calories, 16 grams protein, 1 gram fat, 48 grams carbohydrate, 380 mg sodium, 4 mg cholesterol, 4 percent fat.

B. Breakfast shake: ½ large banana, 1 cup low-fat vanilla yogurt, ¼ cup skim milk, 2 tablespoons oat bran. Mix ingredients in blender on high until blended. Total: about 288 calories, 15 grams protein, 3 grams fat, 47 grams carbohydrate, 181 mg sodium, 12 mg cholesterol, 9 percent fat.

Lunch

Tuna sandwich: Mix 3½ ounces (half a small can) of water-packed tuna (preferably low-salt type) with 2 tablespoons of low-fat cottage cheese (1-percent milkfat only!) and 1 tablespoon of chopped celery (optional: add 1 tablespoon chopped green onion). Serve between 2 slices of whole wheat bread; or, add several lettuce leaves and stuff inside the halves of 1 round of pita bread (6-inch diameter). Whole fresh fruit. Cup of skim milk. Total: about 436 calories, 43 grams protein, 3 grams fat, 59 grams carbohydrate, 550 mg sodium, 69 mg cholesterol, 6 percent fat.

Dinner

Quick Clam Pasta (recipe follows). Cup of skim milk. One-half cup fresh or frozen mixed vegetables (steamed or microwaved, seasoned with lemon juice, pepper; can also use Mrs. Dash Salt-Free Seasoning). Frozen fruit juice bar. Total: about 510 calories, 27 grams protein, 7 grams fat, 86 grams carbohydrate, 190 mg sodium, 62 mg cholesterol, 12 percent fat.

Reminders

■ Coffee, tea or diet pop are optional with all meals, but limit caffeine to two cups coffee or tea, or four 12-ounce cola beverages, per day (you may want to eliminate diet pop, however; research shows aspartame can stimulate appetites).
■ Juice bar limits: 90 calories, 1 gram fat, per bar).
■ Two 80-calorie snacks are allowed per day (See Chapter Two for full list).
■ Don't forget to exercise; by now, beginners should be walking for at least 15 minutes without stopping (see Chapter Five).

*Week II
of the
Dee-troit
Diet*

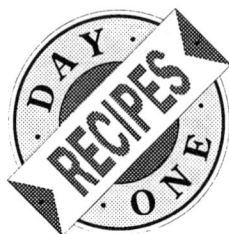

Quick Clam Pasta

2 small cloves garlic, pressed or finely chopped
3 green onions, diced (white and green parts)
1 tablespoon cornstarch
1 6½-ounce can of clams, drained, with liquid
   reserved
2 tablespoons dry white wine (optional)
¼ cup parsley, chopped (or 2 tablespoons
   dried)
2 cups cooked spinach fettuccine or other
   pasta (about 1 cup, or 8 ounces, before
   cooking)

In a non-stick skillet lightly sprayed with cooking oil, saute over
medium heat the garlic and onion for minutes. Meanwhile, put
cornstarch in a bowl. Add clam juice a little at a time, stirring to make a
thin paste. When paste is lump-free, blend rest of clam juice with
cornstarch, then stir in wine. Rinse drained clams in a strainer. Add to
skillet the clams, cornstarch mixture and parsley. Stir and let thicken 1
minute. Divide pasta evenly between 2 plates, and spoon clam sauce
over pasta.
    Makes two servings.
■ **Nutrition details per serving, including wine:** about 286 calories,
16 grams protein, 7 grams fat, 48 grams carbohydrate, 53 mg sodium,
58 mg cholesterol, 22 percent fat.

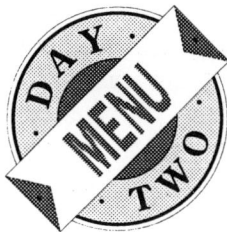

Here are today's approximate nutritional totals, using Breakfast B and not including two 80-calorie snacks: 1,008 calories, 68 grams protein, 15 grams fat, 152 grams carbohydrate, 2,065 mg sodium, 126 mg cholesterol, 13 percent fat.

Breakfast

Choose A or B from Day 1, or choose any breakfast from the Substitute Breakfast page in the Appendix.

Lunch

Fast-food lunch: Wendy's Chili. Fruit side salad (about ¾ cup of mixed sliced fruit; may include watermelon, pineapple, strawberries, peaches, oranges, grapes, honeydew melon, grapefruit and cantaloupe; without dressing). Black coffee, tea or ice water. Total: about 330 calories, 18 grams protein, 8 grams fat, 50 grams carbohydrates, 990 mg sodium, 25 mg cholesterol, 25 percent fat. (Dieters with higher daily calorie allotments can also order a Wendy's plain baked potato, which adds 250 ultra-low-fat calories; request "no butter" added; cut in half if need be to adjust to your daily calorie count; top with chili if desired).

At McDonald's: Oriental Salad with Oriental Dressing (can substitute Light Vinaigrette dressing). Chow mein noodles. Total: about 293 calories, 24 grams protein, 8 grams fat, 29 grams carbohydrate, 606 mg sodium, 94 mg cholesterol, 25 percent fat.

At Hardee's: Seafood salad with Reduced Calorie Italian Dressing (use half of the 2-ounce dressing packet). Total: About 213 calories, 11 grams protein, 7 grams fat, 28 grams carbohydrate, 624 mg sodium, 210 mg cholesterol, 30 percent fat.

Dinner

Frozen chicken dinner. Cup of skim milk. One-half cup steamed

7

*Week II
of the
Dee-troit
Diet*

broccoli or other vegetable, seasoned with lemon juice and pepper or Mrs. Dash salt-free seasoning. Orange or other whole fresh fruit. Total: about 420 calories, 35 grams protein, 4 grams fat, 62 grams carbohydrate, 900 mg sodium, 89 mg cholesterol, 9 percent fat.

Choose a microwave-type or other frozen dinner with no more than 7 grams of fat and 320 calories per serving. Check labels carefully, avoiding those with cream sauces or breading. We used Armour Dinner Classics Lite Chicken Burgundy: 250 calories, 27 grams protein, 4 grams fat, 28 grams carbohydrate, 760 mg sodium, 85 mg cholesterol, 14 percent fat.

Reminders

■ Coffee, tea or diet pop are optional with all meals, but limit caffeine to two cups coffee or tea, or four 12-ounce cola beverages, per day.
■ Two 80-calorie snacks are allowed per day (See Chapter Two for full list).
■ Don't forget to exercise; by now, beginners should be walking for at least 15 minutes without stopping.

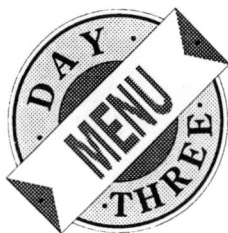

Here are today's approximate nutritional totals, using Breakfast A, and not including two 80-calorie snacks: about 1,065 calories, 61 grams protein, 19 grams fat, 165 grams carbohydrate, 1,195 mg sodium, 121 mg cholesterol, 16 percent fat.

Breakfast

Choose A or B from Day 1, or choose any breakfast from the Substitute Breakfast page in the Appendix.

Lunch

Restaurant sandwich: Sliced turkey (about 2 ounces), lettuce and tomato slices on whole wheat bread, with mustard. Fruit salad without dressing, or small tossed salad dressed with lemon juice. Glass of water. Total: about 325 calories, 15 grams protein, 7 grams fat, 50 grams carbohydrates, 365 mg sodium 47 mg cholesterol, 19 percent fat.

Dinner

Restaurant fish: Five ounces of fish (preferably one high in heart-helping Omega 3 fatty acids, such as salmon, swordfish, snapper, pompano, herring, tuna, mackerel, trout or lake whitefish); order broiled or baked in lemon juice and wine (optional), without butter or other fatty sauce. One-half cup steamed peas or other vegetable, seasoned with lemon juice, pepper and herbs. One small or one-half large plain baked potato, seasoned with lemon juice and pepper (can substitute one-half cup cooked rice, prepared like potato. Small tossed salad dressed with lemon juice or low-calorie Italian dressing (ask for "no-oil" dressing, if available). Total: about 490 calories, 30 grams protein, 11 grams fat, 67 grams carbohydrate, 450 mg sodium, 70 mg cholesterol, 20 percent fat.

7

*Week II
of the
Dee-troit
Diet*

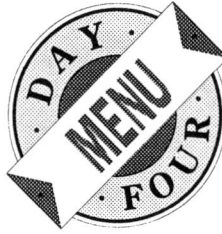

Here are today's approximate nutritional totals, using Breakfast B, and not including two 80-calorie snacks: about 1,108 calories, 58 grams protein, 24 grams fat, 160 grams carbohydrate, 1,800 mg sodium, 50 mg cholesterol, 20 percent fat.

Breakfast

Choose A or B from Day 1, or choose any breakfast from the Substitute Breakfast page in the Appendix.

Lunch

Make-your-own salad from restaurant salad bar, and about 3 tablespoons of low-calorie dressing (see guidelines at the start of this chapter; include lettuce, fresh fruit and vegetables). Two slices of plain bread or 1 large roll (preferably whole wheat). Glass of water. Total: about 300 calories, 7 g protein, 7 g fat, 53 g carbohydrate, 500 mg sodium, 0 mg cholesterol, 21 percent fat.

Dinner

Take-out pizza. Order meatless cheese pizza "with half the cheese"; optional: green pepper, onion and mushroom toppings.

Two slices of a medium or three slices of small pizza. Cup of skim milk. Large tossed salad (1-2 cups lettuce tossed with 1 cup fresh vegetables, such as sliced tomato, cucumber, green pepper and carrot; dress with lemon juice or "no-oil" store-bought salad dressing). Total: about 520 calories, 36 grams protein, 14 grams fat, 60 grams carbohydrate, 1,125 mg sodium, 38 mg cholesterol, 26 percent fat.

Note: At Pizza Hut order Thin 'n Crispy style only, *not* Personal Pan Pizzas. Pizza Hut generally does not deliver, but restaurants have salad bars; order diet pop or ice water in place of skim milk.

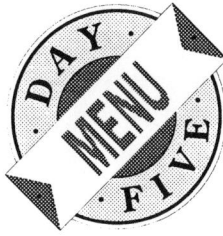

Here are today's approximate nutritional totals, using Breakfast A and Lunch A, and not including two 80-calorie snacks: about 1,143 calories, 62 grams protein, 19 grams fat, 181 grams carbohydrates, 2,380 mg sodium, 82 mg cholesterol, 15 percent fat.

Breakfast

Choose A or B from Day 1, or choose any breakfast from the Substitute Breakfast page in the Appendix.

Lunch

A. Restaurant lunch: bowl (about 12 ounces) of bean or lentil soup, with no meat added; can substitute pea, vegetable or tomato-based soup, including Manhattan clam chowder; avoid cream- or cheese-based soups, and those of meat or poultry broth like chicken noodle). Fruit salad (preferably fresh) without dressing or with packet of "no-oil dressing" brought from home. Slice of bread, small roll or one-half bagel (preferably whole wheat). Total: about 330 calories, 9 grams protein, 7 grams fat, 57 grams carbohydrates, 1,500 grams sodium, 0 grams cholesterol, 19 percent fat.

B. Brown-bag alternative: One plain whole wheat bagel, 1 cup low-sugar low-fat fruit yogurt (no more than 200 calories), fresh carrot. Total: about 400 calories, 16 grams protein, 5 grams fat, 70 grams carbohydrate, 600 mg sodium, 11 mg cholesterol, 11 percent fat.

Dinner

Restaurant chicken: One-half skinless chicken breast (about 3 ounces); order broiled or roasted in lemon juice and wine (optional), without butter or other fatty sauce. One-half cup steamed peas or other vegetable, seasoned with lemon juice, pepper and herbs. One small or

7

*Week II
of the
Dee-troit
Diet*

one-half large plain baked potato, seasoned with lemon juice and pepper (can substitute one-half cup cooked rice). Small tossed salad dressed with lemon juice or low-calorie Italian dressing. Generous scoop (about one-half cup) of orange or lemon sherbet. Total: about 563 calories, 37 grams protein, 11 grams fat, 79 grams carbohydrates, 500 mg sodium, 82 mg cholesterol, 18 percent fat.

Reminders

■ Coffee, tea or diet pop optional with all meals.

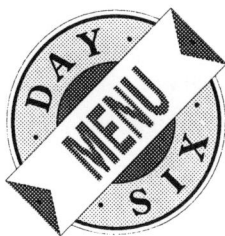

A special note

Today's Dee-troit Diet lunch? A trip to your favorite Chinese restaurant. Oriental fare is a great-tasting way to stoke your personal furnace with complex carbohydrates while you avoid excesses of fat and protein.

Of necessity, Oriental cooks have long learned how to stretch scarce meat and use it as a virtual condiment in tossed dishes of mostly rice and vegetables, minimizing saturated fat and cholesterol. And their primary method of preparation — frying — cuts down on the added fats that food gains from deep frying in cooking oil.

You'll further improve the nutrition score of Oriental restaurant meals by ordering wisely. First, make a few general requests to your waiter or waitress. You'll receive a quick nod or smile of recognition — you aren't the first to ask — for:

■ "No oil" used in stir-frying. Instead, the cook tosses a few tablespoons of water into a steaming wok, searing vegetables and chicken without adding fat calories.

■ "No MSG," or monosodium glutamate. Omitting MSG reduces Oriental cooking's usually excessive sodium content and may help you avoid "Chinese restaurant syndrome," the headaches that sufferers attribute to consuming MSG.

■ "Nothing breaded." Breading absorbs cooking oil and may even mean the food has been deep-fried.

Next, avoid these high-fat traps:

■ Don't order egg drop soup; substitute wonton, sweet and sour, or hot and sour soup.

■ If you order an egg roll, don't eat the fried shell, only the veggies inside.

■ Plum sauce and fried rice are verboten. But thumbs up for hot mustard sauces and plain rice.

7

Week II
of the
Dee-troit
Diet

■ Nix on chow mein noodles, too — a cup has 340 calories.

■ As for good choices? That's easy. Enjoy stir-fried chicken, shrimp or vegetables. Examples abound on any oriental restaurant menu, including gai kow, chicken subgum and good old chop suey. Our favorite? The hot Szechuan-style green beans and rice at Szechuan Garden in Troy, Mich.

Here are approximate nutritional totals for Day 6, using Breakfast B, and not including two 80-calorie snacks: about 1,300 calories, 85 grams protein, 14 grams fat, 206 grams carbohydrate, 2,600 mg sodium, 114 mg cholesterol, 10 percent fat.

Breakfast

Choose A or B from Day 1, or choose any breakfast from the Substitute Breakfast page in the Appendix.

Lunch

Lunch at a Chinese Restaurant (see ordering guidelines above): Bowl of wonton soup. Chicken subgum with one-half cup rice. Tea. One-half fortune cookie. Total: about 520 calories, 42 grams protein, 8 grams fat, 69 grams carbohydrate, 1,100 mg sodium, 78 mg cholesterol, 15 percent fat.

Dinner

Frozen seafood dinner (choose a microwave-type or other frozen fish or chicken dinner with no more than 7 grams of fat and 320 calories per serving; check labels carefully, avoiding those with cream sauces or breading). Cup of skim milk. One-half cup steamed peas or other vegetable, seasoned with lemon juice and pepper or Mrs. Dash salt-free seasoning. Orange or other whole fresh fruit. Frozen fruit juice bar. Total: about 500 calories, 28 grams protein, 3 grams fat, 90 grams carbohydrate, 1,330 mg sodium, 24 mg cholesterol, 5 percent fat.

We used Stouffer's Lean Cuisine Oriental Scallops and Vegetables with Rice (220 calories, 15 grams protein, 3 grams fat, 34 grams carbohydrate, 1,200 mg sodium, 20 mg cholesterol, 12.3 percent fat).

Dinner

■ Coffee, tea or diet pop optional with all meals.

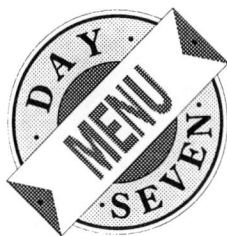

A special note

We'll finish this week of convenience and restaurant meals by spending Day 7 at home, doing just a bit of cooking. Both recipes that follow are a snap, and they make perfect weekend meals.

The whole family will enjoy the dinner recipe for Vegetarian Burritos. At our house, we call 'em by the tongue-in-cheek name my wife, Diana, gave them after she came up with the idea — "Mocko Tacos!"

Here are nutritional totals for Day 7, using Breakfast A and not including two 80-calorie snacks: about 1,170 calories, 69 grams protein, 8 grams fat, 231 grams carbohydrate, 2,200 mg sodium, 13 mg cholesterol, 6 percent fat.

Breakfast

Choose A or B from Day 1, or choose any breakfast from the Substitute Breakfast page in the Appendix.

Lunch

Bowl of asparagus soup (recipe follows). Whole wheat bagel or 2 slices whole wheat toast (spread with 2 tablespoons low-sugar jam or jelly, or apple butter. Cup of skim milk. Tossed salad with slices of hard-boiled egg white and tomato and 2 tablespoons no-oil dressing. Total: about 360 calories, 25 grams protein, 4 grams fat, 85 grams carbohydrates, 750 mg sodium, 5 mg cholesterol, 10 percent fat.

Dinner

Two vegetarian burritos (recipe follows). Cup of skim milk. Whole orange or other fruit. Low-calorie frozen chocolate bar (we used Weight Watchers Double Fudge Artificially Flavored Quiescently Frozen Confection). Total: about 560 calories, 28 grams protein, 3 grams fat, 98 grams carbohydrate, 1,070 mg sodium, 4 mg cholesterol, 5 percent fat.

Week II of the Dee-troit Diet

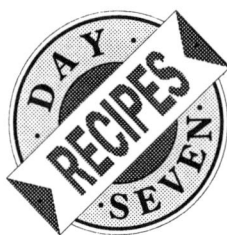

Vegetarian Burritos

1   16-ounce can Heinz Vegetarian Beans (for less sweet taste, use canned red kidney beans)
1   tablespoon plain non-fat yogurt
4   ounces low-sodium V-8 juice
3   small tomatoes (1 chopped)
1   large green pepper
1   whole piece of large whole wheat or rye pita bread (6-7inches in diameter)
¼   cup lettuce, shredded
2   tablespoons green onions, finely sliced
    Mrs. Dash Extra Spicy seasoning

Mash the beans to a paste-like consistency (it's easy if you use an electric mixer or food processor, but it can be done by hand). Mix in yogurt and 1 tablespoon Mrs. Dash Extra Spicy seasoning. Set bean mixture aside.

Make salsa sauce by putting V-8 juice, 2 tomatoes, green pepper and 1 tablespoon of Mrs. Dash Extra Spicy seasoning in blender or food processor. Run at low speed for about 30 seconds (additional Mrs. Dash may be added to taste).

Split pita bread around circumference by working a thumb into the seam, then tearing around the edge. Use one side of a pita slice as a burrito shell. Spread on 4 tablespoons of bean mixture. Sprinkle on shredded lettuce, ½ chopped tomato, green onion and several teaspoons of V-8 salsa sauce. Roll bread like a burrito or fold like a taco to eat (make two for today's dinner).

Serves one (left-over bean mixture will make an additional 5-7 burritos).

■ **Nutrition details per burrito:**about 175 calories, 8 grams protein, 1 gram fat, 33 grams carbohydrate, 450 mg sodium, 0 mg cholesterol.

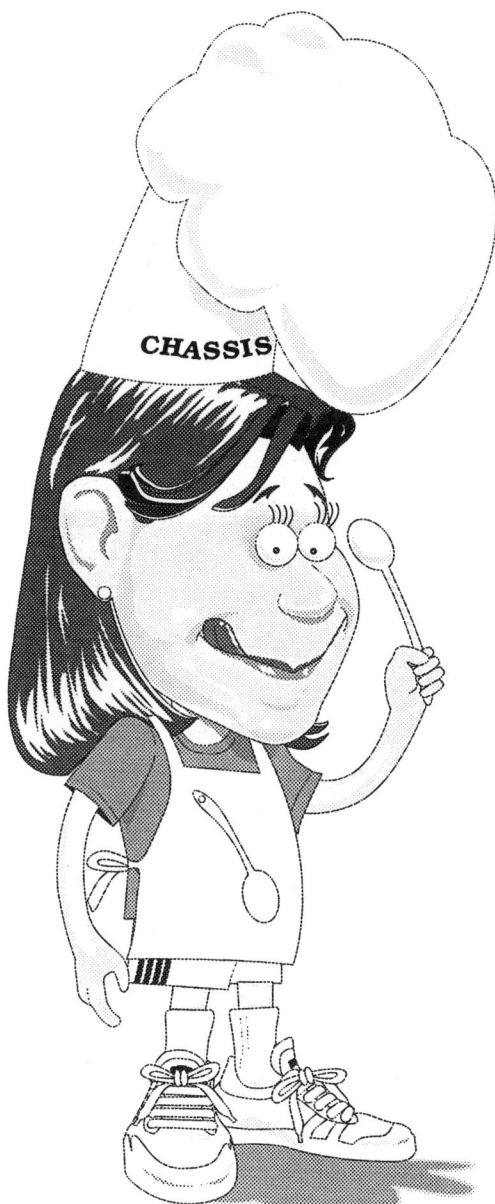

Asparagus Soup

1   10-ounce package of frozen asparagus
    pieces (can substitute broccoli pieces or
    other green vegetable)
1   cup water
1   chicken-flavored bouillon cube (preferably
    low-salt type)
2   tablespoons minced onion flakes (or 1 tea-
    spoon onion powder)
½   cup evaporated skim milk, undiluted
2   tablespoons chopped fresh parsley (or 1
    tablespoon dried parsley)
    Pepper to taste

In a medium-sized saucepan, combine asparagus with water, bouillon
cube and onion flakes. Simmer about 5 minutes. Stir in skim milk,
parsley and pepper. Heat until hot enough to serve, but do not boil. (In
microwave: combine all ingredients in large bowl. Heat on full power for
5 minutes.)

Makes four ½-cup servings.

■ **Nutrition details per serving:** about 55 calories, 5 grams protein,
½ gram fat, 7 grams carbohydrate, 60 mg sodium, 1 mg cholesterol.

8

Week III
of the Dee-troit Diet

Here comes Round Three for getting slim and healthy the smart way, by losing not just weight but *fat* on our low-fat Dee-troit Diet.

This week we'll give you extra tips for accelerating your fat loss by exercising. Increasing your activity level will pay wonderful dividends in improved health and reduced stress, too.

By now we hope you're a regular brisk walker or doing some other steady, uninterrupted activity that qualifies as aerobic exercise. It could be bicycling or stationary cycling, swimming, jogging or cross-country skiing.

If you've neglected to start aerobic exercising, now's a great time. In this chapter we'll pass along workout tips to make walking, or whatever you do, even easier.

(Beginners can take a minute right now to turn back to Chapter Five and read the section "Walk your way to health and weight loss.")

If you've stuck with our beginner's walking schedule, by this time you're on Week III's prescription of 20 minutes daily, five days a week. This is a rewarding week, because somewhere around the 20-minute mark your body's metabolism begins shifting into high-capacity, fat-burning gear. You'll begin to feel more limber and invigorated as you settle into an equilibrium pace that sends a special signal to your body's energy furnace: *Turn on the fat burners.*

At the same time you'll be starting the cardiovascular training effect — the important process of conditioning your heart and lungs to resist aging and heart disease. And you may even feel some mental benefits beginning to kick in as you approach that 20-minute mark; namely, relaxation and stress reduction.

Another special emphasis this week? Improving your cholesterol level. Exercise helps two ways.

First, it helps raise the blood's level of HDL (high-density lipoprotein), or "good" cholesterol. HDL has a protective effect against heart disease.

The threshold for that HDL boost is the equivalent of brisk walking eight to ten miles a week — not much if you spread workouts over three to five sessions.

Second, exercise is also a tremendous help in losing weight. And weight loss generally lowers a high total blood cholesterol level, including the LDL (low-density lipoprotein), or "bad" cholesterol, which clogs arteries and leads to heart attacks and stroke.

We've also included recipes this week that use plenty of legumes, specifically beans and chick peas (also called garbanzos). The special fiber in legumes has been shown to help improve blood cholesterol levels. Our continuing emphasis on seafood helps do the same. So here's to a most healthy Dee-troit Diet week!

(Note: With this week's longer recipes, and your two weeks of Dee-troit Diet experience behind you, we're saving space by not repeating a grocery list here. With this week's somewhat longer recipes, it'll be easier just to take this book with you when you shop.

(Refer back to earlier chapters for everyday needs and check off special needs at each day's recipe listing).

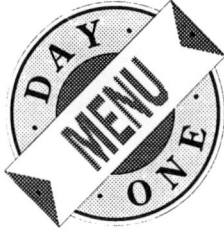

Here are today's approximate nutritional totals, using Breakfast A and not including two 80-calorie snacks: 1,120 calories, 50 grams protein, 5 grams fat, 220 grams carbohydrate, 1,300 mg sodium, 16 mg cholesterol, 4 percent fat.

Breakfast

A. Two eggs whites (or equivalent serving of egg substitute such as Egg Beaters). Prepare soft- or hard-boiled (remove yolks after cooking). Slice of whole wheat toast spread with 2 teaspoons low-sugar jam or jelly (can substitute one-half cup of unsugared dry cereal, such as Post Natural Raisin Bran; maximum of 120 calories and 1 gram of fat per serving; check labels). Cup of skim milk. One-half grapefruit or other whole fresh fruit. Black coffee, tea or ice water. Total: about 250 calories, 16 grams protein, 1 gram fat, 48 grams carbohydrate, 380 mg sodium, 4 mg cholesterol, 4 percent fat.

B. Breakfast shake: ½ large banana, 1 cup low-fat vanilla yogurt, ¼ cup skim milk, 2 tablespoons oat bran. Mix ingredients in blender on high until blended. Total: about 288 calories, 15 grams protein, 3 grams fat, 47 grams carbohydrate, 181 mg sodium, 12 mg cholesterol, 9 percent fat.

Lunch

Large baked potato topped with 3 tablespoons Creamy Low-Cal Dressing (recipe follows) or plain non-fat yogurt. One-half cup of any vegetable, steamed or microwaved (top with 2 tablespoons dressing or plain non-fat yogurt). Whole piece of fresh fruit. Total: about 385 calories, 14 grams protein, 1 gram fat, 80 grams carbohydrate, 233 mg sodium, 5 mg cholesterol, 2 percent fat.

8

Week III of the Dee-troit Diet

Dinner

Serving of Vegetarian Chili (recipe follows). Whole piece of bread or toast or half round of pita bread, preferably whole wheat. Small Tossed Salad topped with 2-3 tablespoons of store-bought no-oil dressing or Creamy Low-Cal Dressing (recipes follow). Cup of skim milk. Baked Apple (recipe follows) or frozen fruit juice bar. Total: about 482 calories, 21 grams protein, 3 grams fat, 92 grams carbohydrate, 660 mg sodium, 7 mg cholesterol, 6 percent fat.

Reminders

■ Coffee, tea or diet pop are optional with all meals. But limit daily caffeine intake to two cups of coffee or strong tea, or four 12-ounce cola beverages (you may want to eliminate diet pop, however; research shows aspartame can stimulate appetites).

■ Two 80-calorie snacks are allowed daily. See list in Chapter Two for suggestions.

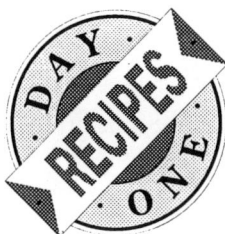

Small Tossed Salad

⅓ medium head lettuce, shredded
⅓ green pepper, sliced
⅓ cup chopped green onion, carrot and celery,
    mixed to taste
2 slices tomato (optional)
¼ cup bean sprouts (optional)

Toss lettuce, green pepper, onion, carrot, celery, and tomato if
desired. Top with bean sprouts, if desired.
Makes one serving.

Creamy Low-Cal Dressing

¼ cup skim milk
1 tablespoon lemon juice
¾ cup low-fat cottage cheese (1-percent milk-
    fat)
½ small onion
1 clove garlic, crushed
½ teaspoon dill weed
    Pepper to taste

Combine ingredients in a blender. Blend on high for 1 minute.
Makes one cup.
■ **Nutrition details per tablespoon:** about 11 calories, 1 gram
protein, less than 1 gram fat, 1 gram carbohydrate, 37 mg sodium, 1 mg
cholesterol, 8 percent fat.

8

*Week III
of the
Dee-troit
Diet*

Vegetarian Chili

½   cup bulgur (see note below)
1   6-ounce can V-8 Juice (preferably low-salt)
½   cup plain non-fat yogurt
1   medium zucchini, chopped
1   medium onion, chopped
1   medium green pepper, chopped
2   cups fresh mushrooms, chopped
1   29-ounce can tomato puree (preferably low-salt; can substitute 4 cups fresh tomatoes, pureed in blender)
1   6-ounce can tomato paste (preferably low-salt)
1   8-ounce can stewed tomatoes (preferably low-salt)
2   15-ounce cans kidney beans
1   teaspoon oregano
½   teaspoon garlic powder
1   teaspoon basil
½   teaspoon chili powder
¼   teaspoon cayenne pepper

Soak bulgur in V-8 for 15 minutes. Add yogurt to mixture and set aside. In a large (at least 4-quart) pot, bottom lightly sprayed with non-stick cooking spray, saute zucchini, onion, green pepper and mushrooms with 2 tablespoons water for several minutes or just until tender. Stir in the bulgur mixture, tomato puree, tomato paste, stewed tomatoes, kidney beans and spices. Cook on medium heat 30-45 minutes.

Serves eight.

■ **Nutrition details per serving:** about 175 calories, 6 grams protein, less than 1 gram fat, 37 grams carbohydrate, 240 mg sodium, 0 mg cholesterol, 3 percent fat.

■ **Note:** Bulgur is also called cracked wheat; we used Hodgson Mill Bulgur Wheat Fortified with Toasted Soy Grits. Cracked wheat is also the main ingredient in tabbouleh mixes, but don't use any accompanying spice packets.

■ **Tip:** this recipe stores well in the refrigerator for a week, far longer in the freezer, and some people say it tastes even better as it ages! The bulgur in the chili looks exactly like bits of ground beef and gives a similar texture. You can make extra and serve it for lunch later in the week (just note the calorie count and substitute).

Baked Apple

1   small apple
½   teaspoon sugar-cinnamon spice (or mix ¼
     teaspoon sugar with ¼ teaspoon cinnamon)
4   "red hot" candies (brands include Cinnamon
     Red Hots and Cinnamon Imperials)

Using a paring knife or apple corer, core apple three-quarters down from stem, removing seeds but taking care not to pierce bottom, so spice flavorings don't leak out. Place sugar-cinnamon spice and "red hots" inside. Put apple on a plate, covering loosely with plastic wrap, and heat on high in microwave oven 2-3 minutes (add 90 seconds for each additional apple); or bake in pre-heated conventional oven at 350 degrees for 20 minutes.
■ **Nutrition details per apple:** about 80 calories, 0 grams protein and fat, 20 grams carbohydrate, trace of sodium, no cholesterol.

8

Plus: The Workout

■ **Aerobic workout:** Continuous walking or stationary cycling for at least 20 minutes. Do it at a comfortable pace but one that makes you breathe deeply. Stop if you feel any pain (and see our cautions in Chapter Five about seeing a doctor before starting to exercise). Slow down if you become uncomfortably fatigued; stop if you feel pain.

■ **Workaday workout:** On your next non-food shopping junket, make a point of wearing comfortable walking shoes. Park where you estimate it will require five minutes of relaxed walking to reach the store. When you leave your car, note the exact time. If you arrive before five minutes is up, stroll past the store and circle back. Use the time to plan your shopping.

■ **Exercise tip:** Hate exercising in the cold? OK, but we bet you dislike those layers of natural insulation you're lugging around even more. Here's a nice thought — If you exercise in cold weather, you'll burn fat faster because just keeping warm takes significant energy.

■ **Life-style tip:** If you're not already wearing your seat belt, start doing so today, not just for safety's sake but for better posture, too. Seat belts, by flattening your spine against the back of a firm car seat, can help prevent or reduce minor low-back pain. But your back won't like being belted to a sponge. If your car seat is mushy, spend $12 to $20 on a special cushion designed to improve lower back support. They're available at many auto and department stores.

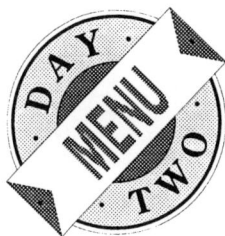

Here are approximate nutritional totals for Day 2, using Breakfast B, and Lunch B, and not including two 80-calorie snacks (see Chapter Two for list): about 1,051 calories, 69 grams protein, 7 grams fat, 176 grams carbohydrate, 2,251 mg sodium, 190 mg cholesterol, 6 percent fat.

Breakfast

Choose A or B from Day 1, or choose any breakfast from the Substitute Breakfast page in the Appendix.

Lunch

A. Bagel and yogurt: Plain, garlic or whole-wheat bagel (or 2 slices whole wheat bread or toast); spread with 1-2 tablespoons low-sugar jam or jelly. One cup low-sugar low-fat fruit yogurt (no more than about 200 calories and 4 grams fat, such as the Dannon "25 percent less sugar" brands). Whole fresh fruit. Total: about 440 calories, 17 grams protein, 5 grams fat, 86 grams carbohydrate, 540 mg sodium, 14 mg cholesterol, 10 percent fat.

B. Bagel and tossed salad with egg: Plain, garlic or whole-wheat bagel (or 2 slices whole wheat bread or toast); spread with 1-2 tablespoons low-sugar jam or jelly. Tossed salad (⅓ head of lettuce; ¼ carrot and ¼ sweet bell pepper, sliced; 2-3 tablespoons no-oil dressing) topped with 1 hard-boiled egg white (remove yolk after cooking). Cup of skim milk. Whole piece of fresh fruit. Total: about 372 calories, 19 grams protein, 2 grams fat, 70 grams carbohydrate, 560 mg sodium, 4 mg cholesterol, 5 percent fat.

Dinner

Serving of Easy Shrimp Creole (recipe follows). One-half cup of cooked rice (enriched white or brown). One-half cup of any fresh or

Week III of the Dee-troit Diet

frozen green vegetable or mixed vegetables (without sauce), steamed or microwaved, and topped with ½ teaspoon Butter Buds Sprinkles (butter flavor seasoning) or lemon juice, and pepper if desired. Small tossed salad (⅓ head of lettuce, topped with ¼ carrot and ¼ sweet bell pepper, sliced; top with 2-3 tablespoons no-oil dressing). Cup of skim milk. Total: about 391 calories, 35 grams protein, 2 grams fat, 59 grams carbohydrates, 1,510 mg sodium, 174 mg cholesterol, 5 percent fat.

Reminders

■ Coffee, tea or diet pop optional with all meals. But don't forget the rules on caffeine and snacks (see Day 1).

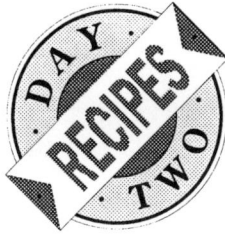

Easy Shrimp Creole

Water
½   cup celery, chopped
½   cup green pepper, finely chopped
½   cup onion, finely chopped
2   tablespoons dry Butter Buds (powdered butter substitute)
2   cloves garlic, finely chopped
1   can tomato sauce (15-ounce, preferably low-salt)
½   teaspoon salt (optional)
¼   teaspoon hot pepper sauce
1   pound medium shrimp, shelled and cleaned
Ground black pepper to taste

Microwave directions: Put ½ cup water, celery, green pepper, onion, Butter Buds and garlic into 2-quart casserole dish with cover. Heat, uncovered, in microwave oven on high 4-5 minutes, until vegetables are tender. Stir in tomato sauce, salt, hot pepper sauce, shrimp and pepper, then heat in microwave oven, covered, for 3 minutes on full power. Set microwave on medium and heat 5 more minutes. Remove and let stand 3 minutes before serving.

To cook on conventional stove: Bring 4 cups of water to boil in a large saucepan. Add shrimp, reducing heat. Simmer for 5 minutes or until shrimp are pink but not tightly curled. Drain immediately and reserve.

In a saucepan, combine ½ cup water, celery, green pepper, onion and garlic. Cook uncovered over medium heat until tender (8-10 minutes). Stir in Butter Buds, tomato sauce, salt, hot pepper sauce and pepper

8

*Week III
of the
Dee-troit
Diet*

until thoroughly mixed. Cook 5 minutes on medium heat. Add shrimp, remove from heat. Let stand 3 minutes before serving.

Serves six.

■ **Nutrition details per serving:** about 122 calories, 20 grams protein, 1 gram fat, 8 grams carbohydrate, 583 mg sodium, 113 mg cholesterol, 7 percent fat.

Plus: The workout

■ **Aerobic workout:** Continuous walking or stationary cycling for at least 20 minutes. Do it at a comfortable pace but one that makes you breathe deeply. Stop if you feel any pain (and see our cautions in Chapter Five about seeing a doctor before starting to exercise); slow down if you become uncomfortably fatigued.

■ **Workaday workout:** When Elisha Otis invented the first safety elevator in 1854, it was a boon to the burgeoning skyline of New York City. But if your midriff is burgeoning, see if your place of employment has that strange architectural feature called *stairs*. But don't dash up and down, then wonder why you're breathless. Tackle steps deliberately, using the break in your routine to unwind or plan part of your day. Naturally, it helps to wear shoes with cushioned soles and low heels.

■ **Life-style tip:** Doing a lot of close work? Manufacturers of computer screens suggest that users take frequent eye breaks. Those who spend hours staring at paperwork or performing other close work — even hobbyists — should do the same. Relaxing your eyes' focusing muscles is as simple as staring off into the distance for several minutes every hour. Start today. Find a window near your work site, then focus on something at least a few hundred yards away for a minute or two. Shift your gaze from near to far several times before going back to work.

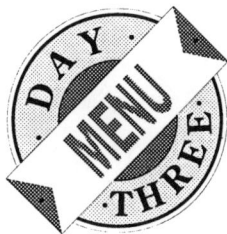

Here are the approximate nutritional totals for Day 3, using Breakfast A, and not including two 80-calorie snacks (see Chapter Two for list): about 1,075 calories, 76 grams protein, 7 grams fat, 180 grams carbohydrate, 2,065 mg sodium, 77 mg cholesterol, 6 percent fat.

Breakfast

Choose A or B from Day 1, or choose any breakfast from the Substitute Breakfast page in the Appendix.

Lunch

Tuna sandwich: Mix 3½ ounces (half a small can) of water-packed tuna (preferably low-salt type) with 2 tablespoons of low-fat cottage cheese (1-percent milkfat only!) and 1 tablespoon of chopped celery (optional: add 1 tablespoon chopped green onion). Serve between 2 slices of whole wheat bread; or add several lettuce leaves and stuff inside the halves of whole round of pita bread (6-inch diameter). Whole fresh fruit. Cup of skim milk. Total: about 436 calories, 43 grams protein, 3 grams fat, 59 grams carbohydrate, 550 mg sodium, 69 mg cholesterol, 6 percent fat.

Dinner

Italian Bean Soup (recipe follows). Slice of whole wheat bread or half round of pita bread. Piece of fresh fruit. Cup of skim milk. Total: about 390 calories, 17 grams protein, 3 grams fat, 73 grams carbohydrate, 1,135 mg sodium, 4 mg cholesterol, 7 percent fat.

8

*Week III
of the
Dee-troit
Diet*

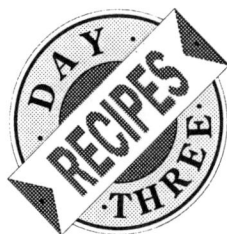

Italian Bean Soup

1   cup dry navy beans
      Water
1   cup chopped onion
1   cup chopped green pepper
2   tablespoons of instant beef bouillon granules
      (preferably low-sodium type)
1   29-ounce can of tomato sauce (preferably
      low-salt type)
1   cup chopped carrot
2   cloves garlic, finely chopped
1½   teaspoons dried basil
1½   teaspoons dried oregano
¼   teaspoon dry mustard powder
½   cup macaroni (preferably whole wheat)

Rinse beans, place in cooking pot and add water to 1 inch above beans. Boil for 2 minutes. Remove from heat, cover and let stand 1 hour. Drain water and add fresh water to 1 inch above beans. Stir in onion, green pepper, bouillon granules, tomato sauce, carrot, garlic, basil, oregano and mustard powder. Cover and simmer 1½ hours. Stir in macaroni and cook uncovered 10-15 minutes.

Makes six hearty servings.

■ **Nutrition details per serving:** about 175 calories, 6 grams protein, 1 gram fat, 35 grams carbohydrate, 850 mg sodium, 0 mg cholesterol, 8 percent fat.

Plus: The workout

■ **Aerobic workout:** If you've exercised briskly two days in a row, today is optional. Relax while you make that delicious bean soup!

■ **Workaday workout:** Turn back the clock on the information age. Try hand-delivering four messages today (perhaps two before lunch, two after). Each should require a minimum stroll of at least 3 minutes. Whether you're letting friends know about neighborhood doings or answering requests from another department at work, you'll burn extra calories while making points for personal contact.

■ **Exercise tip:** Can't see yourself dashing around the local school track or knocking out fast laps in a pool? Don't worry. Exercising at fairly low intensity for long periods is the fastest way to burn off fat, say obesity experts. Why?

In the first 15 minutes of exercising, your muscles are burning mostly glycogen (starch that converts to sugar). After about 20 to 30 minutes of brisk but not exhausting effort, you begin to burn more fat than glycogen. In other words, brisk walking beats sprinting when it comes to winning the battle of the bulge.

8

Week III
of the
Dee-troit
Diet

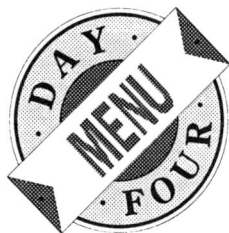

Here are the approximate nutritional totals for Day 4, using Breakfast A, and not including two 80-calorie snacks (see Chapter Two): about 1,045 calories, 60 grams protein, 15 grams fat, 170 grams carbohydrate, 2,140 mg sodium, 73 mg cholesterol, 13 percent fat.

Breakfast

Choose A or B from Day 1, or choose any breakfast from the Substitute Breakfast page in the Appendix.

Lunch

Whole wheat or plain bagel, spread with 1-2 tablespoons of low-sugar jam or jelly. Bean salad, made with ⅓ head lettuce, ¼ cup garbanzo beans (chick peas), ¼ cup bean sprouts (optional), ¼ cup chopped green onion, and 1 sliced hard-boiled egg white, and tossed with 2-3 tablespoons no-oil dressing. Piece of whole fresh fruit. Cup of skim milk. Total: about 410 calories, 24 grams protein, 3 grams fat, 71 grams carbohydrate, 830 mg sodium, 4 mg cholesterol.

Dinner

Quick Skillet Dinner (recipe follows). Small tossed salad (⅓ head of lettuce, topped with ¼ carrot and ¼ sweet bell pepper, sliced; top with 2-3 tablespoons no-oil dressing). Frozen fruit juice bar. Total: about 430 calories, 20 grams protein, 11 grams fat, 61 grams carbohydrate, 940 mg sodium, 65 mg cholesterol, 25 percent fat.

Reminders

■ Coffee, tea or diet pop optional with all meals. But don't forget the rules on caffeine and snacks (see Day 1).

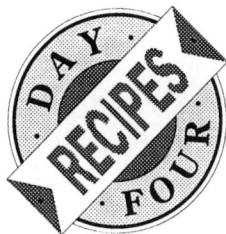

Quick Skillet Dinner

1 cup elbow macaroni (dry)
1 pound ground turkey
1 cup diced onions
1 clove garlic, mashed
   Vegetable oil
1 8-ounce can tomato sauce (preferably low-salt type)
¼-½ teaspoon salt (optional)
¼ teaspoon pepper or to taste
1 cup catsup (preferably low-salt)
1 8-ounce can mushroom stems and pieces, drained
2 tablespoons Worcestershire sauce (can substitute low-salt steak sauce)
½ teaspoons Italian seasoning or low-salt substitute

Cook macaroni in boiling water; drain and set aside. Saute turkey, onions and garlic in a non-stick skillet wiped with vegetable oil, for several minutes until onions are tender. Add tomato sauce, salt, pepper, catsup, mushrooms, Worcestershire sauce and Italian seasoning. Bring to a boil, then simmer gently for about 5 minutes. Add macaroni; simmer 5 minutes more.

Serves six.

■ **Nutrition details per serving:** about 380 calories, 25 grams protein, 11 grams fat, 45 grams carbohydrate, 875 mg sodium, 69 mg cholesterol, 26 percent fat.

8

*Week III
of the
Dee-troit
Diet*

Plus: The workout

■ **Aerobic workout:** Today, beginners are back to at least 20 minutes of continuous brisk walking or stationary cycling at a comfortable pace. Remember, it's much more important to take your time and finish the full 20 minutes than to rush and quit early. But don't be afraid to work up to light perspiration and deep breathing by the time you finish.

■ **Workaday workout:** Take a healthful break from stress. Instead of fighting pressure with tense muscles or tobacco smoke, try this right at your desk or work station. Sit down, close your eyes, then take a deep breath while counting to seven. Exhale slowly through pursed lips; repeat. "As you take in more air, your heart rate slows down and your brain begins to get a better oxygen supply," says psychologist and stress expert Dr. Don Powell of Southfield, Mich., a nationally prominent consultant in employee wellness programs.

■ **Weight-loss tip:** Psychologists and obesity experts say one of the best rewards for a life-style change is charting your progress and watching yourself improve. But the same experts discourage beating a path to the bathroom scale, since rapid weight loss can risk health and is rarely permanent. In addition, novice exercisers may not shed pounds initially, as they change their body composition from unattractive fat to healthy lean weight.

So, instead of daily weigh-ins, try weekly ones. Meantime, check off your progress right on your refrigerator door. Note the exercises you've done and healthful meals eaten. And don't let yourself get hungry. No need to. Each time you eat fresh, unprocessed, complex carbohydrates such as fruit, vegetables and fat-free whole grains, you're unlikely to gain weight. Instead, you're popping nature's own vitamin pills — better than pills, in fact, because research shows that you often benefit more from nutrients in food than in supplements.

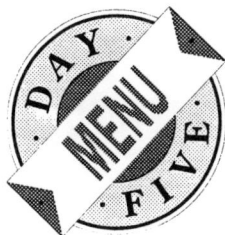

Here are approximate nutritional totals for Day 5, using Breakfast B, and not including two 80-calorie snacks (see Chapter Two): about 1,180 calories, 83 grams protein, 15 grams fat, 177 grams carbohydrate, 1,535 mg sodium, 184 mg cholesterol, 11 percent fat.

Breakfast

Choose A or B from Day 1, or choose any breakfast from the Substitute Breakfast page in the Appendix.

Lunch

Tuna sandwich: Mix 3½ ounces (half a small can) of water-packed tuna (preferably low-salt type) with 2 tablespoons of low-fat cottage cheese (1-percent milkfat only!) and 1 tablespoon of chopped celery (optional: add 1 tablespoon chopped green onion). Serve between 2 slices of whole wheat bread; or, add several lettuce leaves and stuff inside the halves of whole round of pita bread (6-inch diameter). Whole fresh fruit. Cup of skim milk. Total: about 436 calories, 43 grams protein, 3 grams fat, 59 grams carbohydrate, 550 mg sodium, 69 mg cholesterol, 6 percent fat.

Dinner

Light and Lively Eggs (recipe follows; it's great for dinner, ideal for breakfasts or brunch, too). Small tossed salad (⅓ head of lettuce, topped with ¼ carrot and ¼ sweet bell pepper, sliced; top with 2-3 tablespoons no-oil dressing). Piece of fresh fruit. Two pieces of toasted whole wheat bread (if desired, spread with 2 tablespoons low-sugar jam or jelly). Cup of skim milk. Total: about 460 calories, 25 grams protein, 8 grams fat, 73 grams carbohydrate, 805 mg sodium, 103 mg cholesterol, 16 percent fat.

8

Week III of the Dee-troit Diet

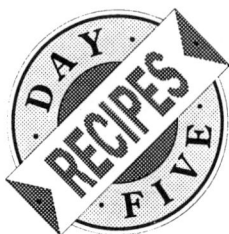

Light and Lively Eggs

5 slices of whole wheat bread
  Vegetable oil
3 whole eggs (large)
6 egg whites (large eggs)
1 tablespoon dry mustard
¾ cup shredded Weight Watchers Natural Part-Skim Milk Cheese or equivalent
½ cup chopped onion
¼ cup finely chopped green pepper
1½ cups skim milk

Cut bread into cubes. Thinly coat inside of 9-by-13-inch pan with vegetable oil; cover bottom with bread cubes. Mix eggs, egg whites, dry mustard, cheese, onion, green pepper and milk. Pour over bread, then refrigerate 2 hours or overnight. Bake 45 minutes at 350 degrees. Let stand for a few minutes, then cut into squares and serve.

Serves six.

■ **Nutrition details per serving:** about 170 calories, 14 grams protein, 6 grams fat, 14 grams carbohydrate, 350 mg sodium, 100 mg cholesterol, 33 percent fat.

Plus: The workout

■ **Aerobic workout:** Beginners should again go for at least 20 minutes of continuous brisk walking or stationary cycling. Go as slow as needed to pace yourself over the full time period.

■ **Workaday workout:** Bushed at work? Instead of collapsing with coffee or a cola while hoping for a lift, try taking a fast five-minute break for calisthenics the way workers do in Japan. Stand up and make like a windmill, first with one arm, then the other. Reach for the sky, then let your arms drop; repeat. Walk briskly in place while you gently punch the air. Breathe deeply. (If your boss can't handle this type of wake-up call, find a rest room or other secluded spot a short stroll away.)

On longer breaks today, beat a path *away* from vending machines, the "snack wagon" or your own kitchen. Try heading out for a five- or ten-minute walk (stairwells are a great escape hatch).

■ **Exercise tip:** Novice exercisers often complain about their feet. Here are ways to pamper your pedal extremities:

☐ Buy a top-quality pair of cushy cotton workout socks. Aww, go ahead — spring for a designer label that only you will see under slacks or sweats. Better yet, check at sports stores for walking styles with special cushioning built in at the heel and ball of the foot.

☐ Don't forget shoes. We know you're smart enough to buy a comfy walking pair. Now, go splurge on a dressy pair with cushioned soles. Many of the new styles could sneak unnoticed into formal offices. Women should check out new styles in cushioned walking pumps.

☐ Give yourself nightly foot massages with a moisturizing lotion, just before retiring. You'll be amazed at the tranquilizing effect.

8

*Week III
of the
Dee-troit
Diet*

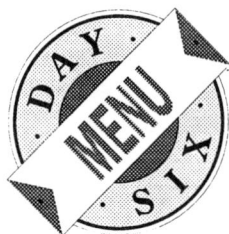

Here are approximate nutritional totals for Day 6, using Breakfast A and Lunch A, and not including two 80-calorie snacks (see Chapter Two): about 1,130 calories, 64 grams protein, 10 grams fat, 207 grams carbohydrate, 1,550 mg sodium, 85 mg cholesterol, 8 percent fat.

Breakfast

Choose A or B from Day 1, or choose any breakfast from the Substitute Breakfast page in the Appendix.

Lunch

A. Bagel and yogurt: Plain, garlic or whole-wheat bagel (or 2 slices whole wheat bread or toast); spread with 1-2 tablespoons low-sugar jam or jelly. One cup low-sugar low-fat fruit yogurt (no more than about 200 calories and 4 grams fat, such as the Dannon "25 percent less sugar" brands). Whole fresh fruit. Total: about 440 calories, 17 grams protein, 5 grams fat, 86 grams carbohydrate, 540 mg sodium, 14 mg cholesterol, 10 percent fat.

B. Bagel and tossed salad with egg: Plain, garlic or whole-wheat bagel (or 2 slices whole wheat bread or toast); spread with 1-2 tablespoons low-sugar jam or jelly. Tossed salad (⅓ head of lettuce; ¼ carrot and ¼ sweet bell pepper, sliced; 2-3 tablespoons no-oil dressing) topped with 1 hard-boiled egg white (remove yolk after cooking). Cup of skim milk. Whole piece of fresh fruit. Total: about 372 calories, 19 grams protein, 2 grams fat, 70 grams carbohydrate, 560 mg sodium, 4 mg cholesterol, 5 percent fat.

Dinner

Broiled Sole with Mustard Dill Sauce (recipe follows). One-half cup fresh or frozen vegetable or mixed vegetables (steamed or microwaved), seasoned with lemon juice and pepper or Mrs. Dash Salt-Free Seasoning. Two boiled new potatoes (or 1 medium regular baked potato, or ¾ cup cooked rice), seasoned with Butter Buds butter substitute and/or Mrs. Dash Salt-Free seasoning. Small Tossed Salad (use Day 1 directions, but try using sliced cucumber and/or radish); top with 2-3 tablespoons store-bought no-oil dressing or leftover Creamy Low-Cal Dressing from Day 1. Total: 437 calories, 31 grams protein, 4 grams fat, 68 grams carbohydrate, 529 mg sodium, 67 mg cholesterol, 8 percent fat.

Reminders

■ Coffee, tea or diet pop optional with all meals. But don't forget the rules on caffeine and snacks (see Day 1).

8

*Week III
of the
Dee-troit
Diet*

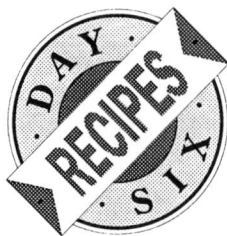

Broiled Sole with Mustard Dill Sauce

1   cup plain non-fat yogurt
2   tablespoons Dijon mustard
¾   teaspoon dried dill weed
     Non-stick cooking spray
2   pounds sole (use four ½-pound fillets or
     more smaller ones; can substitute a similar
     amount of other fish cut into four pieces)

Pre-heat broiler. In small bowl, mix yogurt, mustard and dill weed. Spray broiler rack lightly with cooking spray. Place fish on rack in broiler pan, brushing fillets generously with sauce; place 6 inches from broiler. During cooking, brush on additional sauce once. Turn after 3-5 minutes. Coat other side with sauce, then broil 3 minutes or until fish flakes.
     Serves four.
■ **Nutrition details per serving:** about 135 calories, 21 grams protein, 3 grams fat, 5 grams carbohydrate, 350 mg sodium, 64 mg cholesterol, 21 percent fat.

Plus: The workout

■ **Aerobic workout:** If you're in the mood, go for another minimum 20 minutes of brisk walking or cycling. Alternately, you can take a rest day in our "two days on, one day off" schedule.
■ **Workaday workout:** You say you're *soooo* busy, you just can't leave your desk or the kitchen table? Then stay put! Sit in a sturdy chair (for swivel chairs, use one whose back has at least moderate resistance to flipping backward). With feet together and flat on the floor, grip the front corners of your seat, then exhale as you bring knees toward your chest and return to floor. Work up to 10 or more repetitions.

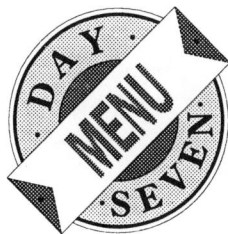

Here are approximate nutritional totals for Day 7, averaging Breakfast A and B, and not including two 80-calorie snacks (see Chapter Two): about 1,200 calories, 79 grams protein, 10 grams fat, 196 grams carbohydrate, 1,360 mg sodium, 101 mg cholesterol, 8 percent fat.

Breakfast

Choose A or B from Day 1, or choose any breakfast from the Substitute Breakfast page in the Appendix.

Lunch

Large baked potato topped with a mixture of 2 tablespoons low-fat cottage cheese, 1 tablespoon chopped onion and 1 tablespoon chopped celery (cottage cheese must be 1-percent milk fat only); or top with ¼ cup reheated Vegetarian Chili (from Day 1 recipe). Piece of fresh fruit. Cup of skim milk. Small tossed salad (⅓ head of lettuce, topped with ¼ carrot and ¼ sweet bell pepper, sliced; top with 2-3 tablespoons no-oil dressing). Total: about 435 calories, 19 grams protein, 1 gram fat, 85 grams carbohydrate, 453 mg sodium, 6 mg cholesterol, 3 percent fat.

Dinner

Chicken Vegetable Skillet Dinner (recipe follows). Small Tossed Salad (use Day 1 directions but try using sliced cucumber and/or radish); top with 2-3 tablespoons no-oil dressing or left-over Creamy Low-Cal Dressing from Day 1. One serving of Low-fat Chocolate Mousse (recipe follows). Total: about 495 calories, 45 grams protein, 7 grams fat, 63 grams carbohydrate, 630 mg sodium, 87 mg cholesterol, 14 percent fat.

Reminders

■ Coffee, tea or diet pop optional with all meals. But don't forget the rules on caffeine and snacks (see Day 1).

8

Week III
of the
Dee-troit
Diet

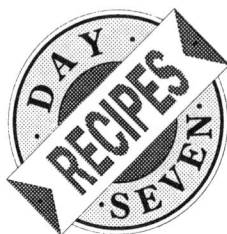

Chicken Vegetable Skillet

1   10-ounce package frozen broccoli (can sub-
    stitute any green vegetable or mixed vege-
    tables)
1   cup uncooked white or brown rice
2   8-ounce whole chicken breasts — skinned,
    boned and cut into ½-inch strips
¼   cup onion, chopped
2   tablespoons liquid Butter Buds (powdered
    butter substitute mixed with water)
1   teaspoon lemon juice (fresh juice tastes
    noticeably better but can use reconstituted)
¼   teaspoon each, garlic powder and onion
    powder
3   medium tomatoes, cut into wedges

Allow broccoli to begin thawing. Prepare rice according to package
directions, except use no margarine and cut cooking time in half (do not
drain). In non-stick skillet sprayed with cooking spray, over medium
heat, cook chicken strips and onion, using a dash of liquid Butter Buds or
water to prevent sticking. Stir continuously. Cook 3-5 minutes. Add rice
and its cooking water. Add broccoli, lemon juice, garlic powder and onion
powder. Simmer covered 10-12 minutes or until rice is tender. Arrange
tomato wedges on top, cover and simmer another 2 minutes.
    Makes four 1¼-cup servings.
■ **Nutrition details per serving:** about 400 calories, 42 grams
protein, 6 grams fat, 45 grams carbohydrate, 112 mg sodium, 85 mg
cholesterol, 14 percent fat.

Low-Fat Chocolate Mousse

1   1.7-ounce packet of instant sugar-free pud-
    ding mix, chocolate or chocolate fudge
2   cups skim milk
4   tablespoons Cool Whip Extra Creamy Dairy
    topping

In medium-size mixing bowl, place pudding mix and skim milk. Whip with blender on medium speed for 45 seconds. Add Cool Whip and whip 30 seconds. Refrigerate at least 15 minutes.

Serves six.

■ **Nutrition details per serving:** about 45 calories, 3 grams protein, 1 gram fat, 6 grams carbohydrate, 110 mg sodium, 2 mg cholesterol, 20 percent fat.

Plus: The workout

■ **Aerobic workout:** Resume or continue uninterrupted brisk walking or stationary cycling for at least 20 minutes. If you're bored, get a friend to join you or strap on earphones from a portable cassette player/radio.

■ **Workaday workout:** Learn to build minutes of calorie-burning activity into your everyday life. The easiest way is by walking to accomplish an errand. The destination gives purpose to your walk. Today, think of one or two small items — perhaps toiletries or camera film — available at a shop near you. If necessary, drive your car to within walking distance and park. Then hoof it to the store. (You could spend those moments thinking about how little of your life you spend walking compared with our ancient ancestors, who spent most of their waking hours walking in search of food.)

■ **Life-style tip:** Physiologists say most people become highly depen-
dent on one side of the body, usually the right. For those doing prolonged tasks, that leads to excessive fatigue and unnecessary muscle strain, particularly in the neck, shoulder and arm. You can eliminate much of this fatigue by splitting tasks with both sides of your body. That means switching hand positions when shoveling snow, digging in the garden, painting, washing, even brushing your teeth.

8

*Week III
of the
Dee-troit
Diet*

At first, you'll have to slow down and let the less-used hand do a sometimes awkward job for you (you can then empathize with small children and stroke patients). After practice, however, you may be surprised at how quickly a jolt to the sleeping half of your body wakens latent ambidexterity.

9

Week IV
of the Dee-troit Diet

Everyone is used to nutritional avoidance therapy — don't eat this, don't eat that — to lose weight and improve cholesterol levels.

But science is just beginning to learn about foods everyone *should* eat, foods that help people shed weight and have better than a neutral effect on cholesterol — they actually improve cholesterol levels in the blood.

This week Dee-troit Dieters are getting such foods as oat bran muffins for breakfast, citrus fruit for lunch and ocean fish for dinner. All have beneficial effects on the levels of fats in the blood, fats that profoundly affect our health.

Not surprisingly, cholesterol-fighting food *doesn't* include cheeseburgers, french fries and milk shakes. It does include food with a certain kind of dietary fiber, the non-nutritive material our grandparents called "roughage," abundant in fresh fruit, vegetables and whole grains, which is often milled away from processed and fast foods.

Dietary fiber gained attention early in the 1980s when nutritionists realized its value in preventing digestive ailments, ranging from constipation and hemorrhoids to more serious diseases such as diverticulosis and colon cancer. Fiber is thought to expand in the intestines, preventing the compaction of waste matter and speeding the exit of noxious, even cancer-causing compounds.

Researchers learned that fiber comes in two types. The type most beneficial to digestion is insoluble fiber. Whole wheat bread is a good source. A second type, soluble fiber, helps shunt damaging cholesterol from the body, although theorists are still unsure how that occurs.

Food high in soluble fiber includes oat bran (the husk of milled oats); legumes like kidney beans; and fruit, including grapefruit, oranges, apples, grapes and prunes. Cholesterol experts recommend eating a variety of soluble fiber sources, which is why we've included many in this book's menus.

Oat bran has gotten most of the attention because it has a proven effect and is easy to add to food such as baked goods, pancakes, breakfast cereal and muffins. How much should you get?

Those with serious cholesterol problems may want to heed the prescription from the University of Kentucky at Lexington, where researchers found that half a cup daily caused an 8-10 percent drop in total cholesterol, and a larger drop in the damaging LDL-type cholesterol.

For the average person, we suggest sprinkling a couple of tablespoons on breakfast cereal. Note that our breakfast shakes specifically call for oat bran.

Oat bran is sold in virtually all health food stores and in a growing number of supermarkets. Along with other brands, many supermarkets are beginning to stock one of two identical Quaker products: Mother's Oat Bran Creamy High-Fiber Hot Cereal, and Quaker Oat Bran Creamy High-Fiber Hot Cereal.

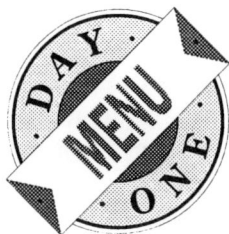

These are approximate nutritional totals for Day 1, averaging lunch choices and not including two 80-calorie snacks: about 1,190 calories, 80 grams protein, 11 grams fat, 191 grams carbohydrate, 1,400 mg sodium, 145 milligrams cholesterol, 8 percent fat.

Breakfast

Three-quarters cup of Post Natural Raisin Bran or serving of other unsweetened dry cereal (maximum of 120 calories and 1 gram of fat per serving; check labels). Slice 1 banana over cereal, or eat separately 1 banana or other whole fresh fruit (or half grapefruit). Cup of skim milk (or 8 ounces plain non-fat yogurt). Total: about 290 calories, 11 grams protein, 1 grams fat, 59 grams carbohydrate, 300 mg sodium, 4 mg cholesterol, 3 percent fat.

Brunch

A. At home: Serving of Egg White Omelet (recipe follows). Two slices of bread, toasted, preferably whole wheat; spread with 2 tablespoons low-sugar jam or jelly. One orange or other whole fresh fruit (or half grapefruit). Cup of skim milk. Total: about 435 calories, 22 grams protein, 8 grams fat, 68 grams carbohydrate, 575 mg sodium, 110 mg cholesterol, 17 percent fat.

B. At a restaurant: Elias Bros. Big Boy Vegetarian Egg Beater Omelet (made with Egg Beaters egg substitute, green pepper and mushroom, topped with tomato slices). With 2 slices plain toast spread with low-cal preserve. Bowl of sliced bananas or strawberries. Glass of skim milk (10 ounces). Total: about 470 calories, 28 grams protein, 6 grams fat, 77 grams carbohydrate, 535 mg sodium, 6 mg cholesterol, 12 percent fat.

9

Week IV of the Dee-troit Diet

Dinner

Four ounces of Easy Skinless Chicken (recipe follows; 4 ounces of chicken prepared this way has the approximate volume of 1⅓ pieces sandwich bread). One-half cup of any fresh or frozen green vegetable or mixed vegetables (without sauce), steamed or microwaved, topped with ½ teaspoon Butter Buds Sprinkles (butter-flavored seasoning) or lemon juice, and pepper if desired. Medium baked potato, served with ½ teaspoon Butter Buds sprinkles (or teaspoon of liquefied Butter Buds powdered mix) or Molly McButter Sprinkles (All-Butter flavor, or Sour Cream and Butter flavor). Small Tossed Salad (recipe follows), topped with 3 tablespoons store-bought "no-oil" dressing. Legal Chocolate Ice Cream Soda (recipe follows). Total: about 500 calories, 45 grams protein, 5 grams fat, 70 grams carbohydrate, 640 mg sodium, 95 mg cholesterol, 9 percent fat.

Reminders

■ Coffee, tea or diet pop are optional with all meals, but limit caffeine intake to two cups coffee or tea or four 12-ounce cola beverages per day (you may want to eliminate diet pop; research shows aspartame can stimulate appetites).
■ Two 80-calorie snacks are allowed per day. Use extra snacks or adjust meal portion sizes to achieve a daily calorie count that's right for your target weight (multiply target weight by 10; but if you're hungry, eat more of the legal snacks).
■ Don't forget to exercise.

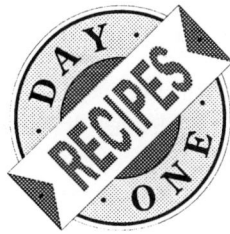

Egg White Omelet

1   teaspoon vegetable oil (preferably canola oil, such as Puritan brand)
½   cup chopped onion (about 1 whole medium onion or ⅓ large onion)
¼   cup chopped green pepper (about ½ pepper)
½   cup sliced mushrooms (about 4 large mushrooms; or substitute 4-ounce can sliced mushrooms)
4   egg whites, 1 yolk (large eggs)

Place oil in the middle of a large non-stick skillet (lined with Teflon or equivalent) over medium high heat. Saute onion in pan 2-3 minutes, moving it around in the oil with a spatula. Add green pepper and mushrooms; saute additional 2-3 minutes, reducing heat to medium. While vegetables are cooking, place 4 egg whites in a large mixing bowl. Whip whites briskly for 1 minute. Then add yolk and blend thoroughly. Using spatula, distribute vegetables fairly evenly around skillet, then pour in egg mixture. Allow to cook 3-4 minutes, until sides of omelet begin curling and top is mostly dry. Go around rim of pan with spatula to loosen omelet, then ease spatula under one side of omelet and flip it onto the other side, leaving half a circle of egg. Remove from heat and serve immediately; or wait 1 minute for a firmer omelet.

Serves two.

■ **Nutrition details per serving:** about 118 calories, 9 grams protein, 6 grams fat, 7 grams carbohydrate, 100 mg sodium, 105 mg cholesterol, 42 percent fat.

9

Week IV of the Dee-troit Diet

Easy Skinless Chicken

Start with 1 large roasting chicken (a 6-pound chicken provides several dinner servings and leaves leftover portions that become sandwiches or salads later in the week; for Day 7 dinner, which serves four, freeze ½-pound — about the volume of 2½ slices of sandwich bread).

Use a very large pot for boiling, about 8- to 10-quart capacity. Fill with about 6 quarts water, enough to cover chicken completely and leave 1 inch of water above it (immerse chicken to be sure). Over high heat, bring water to a full boil. Put chicken in pot. When water stops boiling (about 5 seconds) remove chicken, using tongs or meat fork. Place chicken on a plate while bringing water to full boil a second time. Return chicken to pot. Cover and turn off heat. Leave chicken in pot at least 1 hour. To serve, remove chicken from pot and remove skin. It will pull off easily, taking with it most of the fat. Skim fat off stock and reserve for making soup if desired (note: bottom third of stock pot contains richest stock; unless you need soup for the entire neighborhood you can pour off the top two-thirds of liquid).

■ **Nutrition details per 4-ounce serving:** about 172 calories, 33 grams protein, 3 grams fat, 0 grams carbohydrate, 72 mg sodium, 88 mg cholesterol.

Small Tossed Salad

⅓ medium head lettuce, shredded
⅓ green pepper, sliced
⅓ cup chopped green onion, carrot and celery, mixed to taste
2 slices tomato (optional)
¼ cup bean sprouts (optional)

Toss lettuce, green pepper, onion, carrot, celery, and tomato, if desired. Top with bean sprouts, if desired.

Serves one.

■ **Nutrition details per serving:** about 40 calories, 2 grams protein, 0 grams fat, 8 grams carbohydrate, 35 mg sodium, 0 mg cholesterol (for tomato and sprouts, add 15 calories).

Legal Chocolate Ice Cream Soda

2 ounces Weight Watchers Chocolate Fudge
Ice Milk (about 1 ice cream scoop's-worth or
rounded scoop with soup spoon).

6 ounces Canfield's Diet Chocolate Fudge
soda (½ can)

Place ice milk in clear glass. Pour soda over it. Enjoy with straw and
spoon.

Serves one.

■ **Nutrition details per serving:** about 57 calories, 2 grams protein, 1
gram fat, 9 grams carbohydrate, 80 mg sodium, 4 mg cholesterol, 23
percent fat.

9

*Week IV
of the
Dee-troit
Diet*

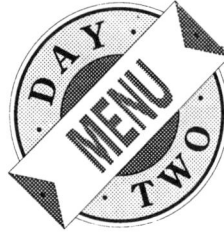

These are approximate nutritional totals for Day 2, averaging breakfast and lunch choices (not including two 80-calorie snacks — see list in Chapter Two): about 1,200 calories, 71 grams protein, 18 grams fat, 190 grams carbohydrate, 3,050 mg sodium, 165 mg cholesterol, 18 percent fat.

Breakfast

Choose A, B or C, or choose any breakfast from the Substitute Breakfast page in the Appendix.

A. Two egg whites, or equivalent serving of egg substitute such as Egg Beaters (soft- or hard-boil whole eggs, removing yolks after cooking). Slice of whole wheat toast spread with 1 tablespoon low-sugar jam or jelly (can substitute one-half cup of unsugared raisin bran, such as Post Natural Raisin Bran). Cup of skim milk or plain non-fat yogurt. One orange or other whole fresh fruit (or half grapefruit). Total: about 250 calories, 16 grams protein, 1 gram fat, 48 grams carbohydrate, 380 mg sodium, 4 mg cholesterol, 4 percent fat.

B. Breakfast shake: ½ large banana, 1 cup low-fat vanilla yogurt, ¼ cup skim milk, 2 tablespoons oat bran. Mix ingredients in blender on high until blended. Total: about 288 calories, 15 grams protein, 3 grams fat, 47 grams carbohydrate, 181 mg sodium, 12 mg cholesterol, 9 percent fat.

C. Two Duncan Hines Oat Bran and Honey muffins (from mix using egg whites only; 12 muffins per mix; this mix was lowest in fat and highest in cholesterol-lowering fiber of mixes and ready-made brands we checked). Half-cup skim milk or plain non-fat yogurt. One orange or other whole piece fresh fruit (or half grapefruit). Total: about 330, 7 grams protein, 7 grams fat, 59 grams carbohydrate, 390 mg sodium, 2 mg cholesterol, 19 percent fat.

Lunch

A. Country Chicken Sandwich: 2-ounce slice of skinless chicken or turkey (you can use leftover chicken, preferably white meat, from Day 1; 2 ounces of chicken or turkey almost exactly covers a piece of sandwich bread with meat that is about half as thick as the bread). Serve between 2 slices of whole wheat bread or inside 1 whole round of pita bread (6-inch diameter); spread with 2 tablespoons plain non-fat yogurt; serve with with lettuce leaves and one-half sliced tomato. Cup of skim milk. Whole fresh fruit. Optional: slice of onion for sandwich. Total: about 420 calories, 32 grams protein, 5 grams fat, 63 grams carbohydrate, 510 mg sodium, 48 mg cholesterol, 11 percent fat.

B. Sub Shop Lunch: Eight-Inch Tubby's Turkey Sub Sandwich (request "no cheese or mayonnaise") or similar sandwich with roll, lettuce, onion, tomato and turkey, but *without* red meat, cheese, mayonnaise or butter); ask for a packet (1¾-ounce) of Tubby's Light Italian Dressing, for spreading inside sandwich. Tubby's 8-ounce Tomato Florentine soup (request "no crackers" with soup; can substitute Chicken Noodle soup). Ice water. Total: about 470 calories, 28 grams protein, 11 grams fat, 63 grams carbohydrate, 2,500 mg sodium, 67 mg cholesterol, 21 percent fat.

Dinner

Frozen dinner. Choose a microwave-type or other frozen dinner with no more than 7 grams of fat and 320 calories per serving; check labels carefully, avoiding those with cream sauces or breading. We chose Le Menu LightStyle Veal Marsala with vegetable-rice medley: about 260 calories, 20 grams protein, 6 grams fat, 31 grams carbohydrates, 800 mg sodium, 100 mg cholesterol, 21 percent fat.

Serve with: Slice of whole wheat bread or one-half cup additional cooked rice (you can spread 1 tablespoon of low-sugar jam or jelly on the bread; top rice with 1 tablespoon of store-bought "no-oil" dressing, or use Butter Buds butter substitute or Mrs. Dash Salt-Free seasoning); Small Tossed Salad (see recipe after Day 1 menu) with 2 tablespoons "no-oil" dressing or use Low-Cal Dressing (recipe follows); frozen fruit juice bar (juice bar limit: 90 calories, 1 gram fat). Total: about 490 calories, 26 grams protein, 8 grams fat, 79 grams carbohydrate, 1,275 mg sodium, 100 mg cholesterol, 15 percent fat.

9

Week IV
of the
Dee-troit
Diet

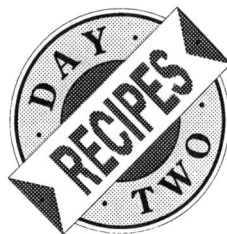

Creamy Low-Cal Dressing

¼   cup skim milk
1   tablespoon lemon juice
¾   cup low-fat cottage cheese (1-percent milk-
    fat)
½   small onion
1   clove garlic, crushed
½   teaspoon dill weed
    Pepper to taste

Combine ingredients in a blender. Blend on high for 1 minute.
Makes one cup.

■ **Nutrition details per tablespoon:** about 11 calories, 1 gram
protein, less than 1 gram fat, 1 gram carbohydrate, 37 mg sodium, 1 mg
cholesterol, 8 percent fat.

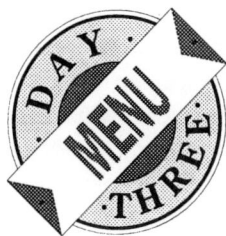

These are approximate nutritional totals for Day 3, averaging breakfast choices and dinner choices and using Lunch B (not including two 80-calorie snacks): about 1,225 calories, 40 grams protein, 11 grams fat, 232 grams carbohydrate, 2,230 mg sodium, 18 mg cholesterol, 8 percent fat.

Breakfast

Choose A or B from Day 2, or choose any breakfast from the Substitute Breakfast page in the Appendix.

Lunch

A. Restaurant salad bar with soup.

At Bonanza Family Restaurants Freshtastics Food Bar, make yourself a large salad of lettuce and cabbage leaves, topped with your choice of mushrooms (whole or sliced, not mushrooms in sauce), peas, carrots, chick peas (garbanzo beans), cucumbers, green pepper, bean sprouts, broccoli, cauliflower, radish, celery, onion and beets (no chopped egg, cheese or meat, and no croutons or bacon bits). Dress with 2-3 ladles of Low-Calorie Italian Dressing (you may have to request it if you don't see it). Dinner roll without butter. One cup Garden Vegetable soup. Three heaping serving spoonfuls of bite-size pretzels. Ice Water. Total, about 435 calories, 11 grams protein, 12 grams fat, 85 grams carbohydrate, 2,500 mg sodium, trace of cholesterol, 25 percent fat.

At Elias Bros. Big Boy, order soup, salad bar and fruit from the Health Smart menu. Make large salad as in Bonanza listing. Dress with 2-3 ladles of Buttermilk Dressing. Bowl of cabbage soup. Two slices whole wheat bread. Bowl of sliced strawberries or bananas. Cup of skim milk. Total: about 480 calories, 22 grams protein, 11 grams fat, 74 grams carbohydrate, 1,580 mg sodium, 26 mg cholesterol, 21 percent fat.

9

Week IV of the Dee-troit Diet

B. Make your own salad and canned soup. One 8-ounce bowl of non-cream base meatless vegetable or tomato soup, made without milk (preferably low-salt type; check label: no more than 2 grams of fat per 4-ounce serving). Large tossed salad (make as in Bonanza restaurant listing), topped with 2-3 tablespoons of store-bought "no-oil" dressing. Slice of bread or toast (preferably whole wheat; tablespoon of low-sugar jam or jelly is optional). Scoop of orange or lemon sherbet (quarter cup; 70-calorie serving). Cup of skim milk. Total: about 435 calories, 15 grams protein, 6 grams fat, 81 grams carbohydrate, 800 mg sodium, 8 mg cholesterol, 12 percent fat.

Dinner

A. Wendy's Super Bar meatless tomato sauce with vegetables and pasta. Order Super Bar and ice water. Serve yourself the following: Tossed salad of lettuce and vegetables (but no cheese, egg, bacon bits or olives), topped with 2 ladles of Reduced Calorie Italian Dressing; return to Super Bar for 5 heaping ladles of Pasta Medley (pasta with vegetables), topped with 3-4 ladles of Meatless Tomato Sauce; return to Super Bar for fresh fruit dessert (up to 1 cup of sliced fruit). Total: about 520 calories, 15 grams protein, 4 grams fat, 106 grams carbohydrate, 1,770 mg sodium, 0 mg cholesterol, 7 percent fat.

B. At-home meatless spaghetti: Two-thirds cup of Meatless Spaghetti Sauce (recipe follows), poured over 1 cup of cooked spaghetti or other pasta. Small Tossed Salad (see Day 1 recipe), topped with 3 tablespoons of store-bought "no-oil" dressing or Creamy Low-Cal Dressing (see Day 2 recipe). Cup of skim milk. Frozen fruit juice bar. Total: about 520 calories, 24 grams protein, 2 grams fat, 100 grams carbohydrate, 530 mg sodium, 3 mg cholesterol, 3 percent fat.

Reminders

■ Coffee, tea or diet pop are optional with all meals, but limit caffeine intake to two cups coffee or tea or four 12-ounce cola beverages per day (you may want to eliminate diet pop; research shows aspartame can stimulate appetites).

■ Two 80-calorie snacks are allowed per day. Use extra snacks or adjust meal portion sizes to achieve a daily calorie count that's right for your target weight (multiply target weight by 10; but if you're hungry, eat more of the legal snacks).

■ Don't forget to exercise.

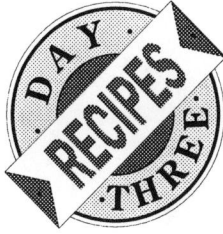

Meatless Spaghetti Sauce

1   teaspoon olive oil
1   large onion, chopped (or 1 cup frozen chopped onion)
2   cloves garlic, minced (optional)
1   cup diced green pepper (fresh or frozen)
¾   cup finely sliced mushrooms (or 4-ounce can)
1   28-ounce can of tomatoes with juice or puree (preferably low-salt type)
1   6-ounce can of tomato paste
1   teaspoon Italian seasoning
¼   teaspoon black pepper

Place oil in a large non-stick skillet or saucepan. Saute onion and garlic over medium heat until translucent (2-3 minutes). Add green pepper and mushrooms and continue cooking 2 minutes, stirring often. Add tomatoes and their liquid, breaking with wooden spoon into small chunks. Add tomato paste, water, Italian seasoning and black pepper. Bring to boil over medium heat. Reduce heat to low and let sauce simmer with cover cracked open to let steam escape, stirring occasionally (reduce heat if sauce sticks to pan bottom). Cook until thickens (about 10-15 minutes).

Serves six.

■ **Nutrition details per ⅔ cup serving:** about 105 calories, 3 grams protein, 1 gram fat, 23 grams carbohydrate, 252 mg sodium, 0 mg cholesterol, 9 percent fat.

9

*Week IV
of the
Dee-troit
Diet*

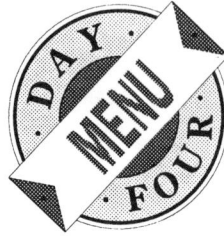

These are approximate nutritional totals for Day 4, averaging choices for breakfast, lunch and dinner, but not including two 80-calorie snacks: about 1,280 calories, 79 grams protein, 19 grams fat, 199 grams carbohydrate, 3,680 mg sodium, 139 mg cholesterol, 13 percent fat.

Breakfast

Choose A or B from Day 2, or choose any breakfast from the Substitute Breakfast page in the Appendix.

Lunch

A. Burger King lunch: Chicken Salad with packet of Reduced Calorie Italian Dressing. Vegetarian Whopper (order without meat and mayonnaise), ordered with extra packet of Reduced Calorie Italian Dressing. Ice Water. Spread about half of a dressing packet (to taste) inside the Whopper. Use remaining dressing on salad. Total: about 445 calories, 27 grams protein, 12 grams fat, 60 grams carbohydrate, 2,800 mg sodium, 50 mg cholesterol, 24 percent fat. (Note: a Vegetarian Whopper, ordered without meat or mayonnaise, is tasty and filling yet contains only 247 calories and 4 grams of fat.)

B. At-home lunch: Easy Chicken Salad. Start with about one-half head of lettuce. Crumble in large bowl. Top with about 1 cup of mixed, sliced vegetables of your choosing. That may include cabbage, green pepper, mushroom, peas, carrot, cucumber, tomato, bean sprouts, broccoli, cauliflower, radish, celery, onion or beets. Add 2 ounces of skinless cooked chicken, cut or torn into small pieces. Toss with 5 tablespoons store-bought "no-oil" dressing. Serve with piece of bread or toast, or pita bread (preferably whole wheat; serve plain or spread with 1 tablespoon low-sugar jam or jelly). Cup of skim milk. Whole piece of fresh fruit. Total: about 440 calories, 30 grams protein, 4 grams fat, 71 grams carbohydrate, 570 mg sodium, 48 mg cholesterol, 8 percent fat.

Dinner

A. Chinese restaurant: Stir-fried shrimp with vegetables and rice (or, for even less fat, order hot 'n spicy Szechuan-style vegetarian green beans and rice; in either case, request "No oil" used in stir frying; instead, the cook tosses spoonfuls of water into a steaming wok to sear food). Eaten with about ¾ cup rice and bowl of wonton soup. Tea. One fortune cookie. Total: about 600 calories, 37 grams protein, 11 grams fat, 90 grams carbohydrate, 2,200 mg sodium, 100 mg cholesterol, 17 percent fat. (Note: reduce sodium by requesting food prepared "without MSG.")

B. At home: Frozen seafood dinner. Choose a microwave-type or other frozen dinner with no more than 7 grams of fat and 320 calories per serving; check labels carefully. Two we liked were Mrs. Paul's Fish Florentine and Mrs. Paul's Fish Dijon with Asparagus. Serve with rice (about ½ to ¾ cup cooked); and Small Tossed Salad (see Day 1 recipe), topped with 3 tablespoons store-bought "no-oil" dressing. Cup of skim milk. Frozen fruit juice bar. Total: about 550 calories, 38 grams protein, 7 grams fat, 82 grams carbohydrate, 1,200 mg sodium, 64 mg cholesterol, 12 percent fat.

Reminders

■ Coffee, tea or diet pop are optional with all meals, but limit caffeine intake to two cups coffee or tea or four 12-ounce cola beverages per day (you may want to eliminate diet pop; research shows aspartame can stimulate appetites).

■ Two 80-calorie snacks are allowed per day. Use extra snacks or adjust meal portion sizes to achieve a daily calorie count that's right for your target weight (multiply target weight by 10; but if you're hungry, eat more of the legal snacks).

■ Don't forget to exercise.

9

*Week IV
of the
Dee-troit
Diet*

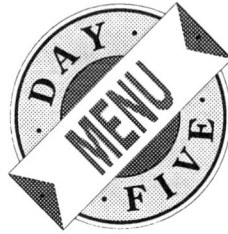

These are approximate nutritional totals for Day 5, averaging breakfast choices, with Lunch A and the scallops dinner (not including two 80-calorie snacks): 1,180 calories, 56 grams protein, 8 grams fat, 226 grams carbohydrate, 1,720 milligrams sodium, 46 milligrams cholesterol, 6 percent fat.

Breakfast

Choose A or B from Day 2, or choose any breakfast from the Substitute Breakfast page in the Appendix.

Lunch

A. Bagel and yogurt lunch. Plain, garlic or whole-wheat bagel (or two slices whole wheat bread or toast); spread with 1-2 tablespoons low-sugar jam or jelly. One cup low-sugar low-fat fruit yogurt (no more than about 200 calories and 4 grams fat, such as the Dannon "25 percent less sugar" brands). Medium-size fresh carrot and stalk celery, cut into strips. Total: about 440 calories, 17 grams protein, 5 grams fat, 86 grams carbohydrate, 540 mg sodium, 14 mg cholesterol, 10 percent fat.

B. Kentucky Fried Chicken lunch. Order ala carte: one 4-ounce cup of baked beans, one 4-ounce cup of mashed potatoes (specify "without gravy"; can substitute additional cup of potatoes for beans); one corn on the cob (specify "without butter"); one Original Recipe "center breast"; ice water. Using plastic fork supplied with order, remove chicken skin and do *not* eat (be sure to request "Wet Naps" for hands clean-up). Total, about 475 calories, 47 grams protein, 6 grams fat, 58 grams carbohydrate, 820 mg sodium, 91 mg cholesterol, 11 percent fat.

Dinner

Start preparation at least 8 hours ahead; you can substitute Lunch B.

for this dinner if you had Lunch A.

One Seafood Kebab (recipe follows). Rice (about ½ cup cooked rice; season with Mrs. Dash Salt-Free Lemon & Herb seasoning, Butter Buds sprinkles (butter-flavor seasoning), and pepper to taste. Small Tossed Salad (see Day 1 recipe), topped with with 3 tablespoons store-bought "no-oil" dressing. Cup of skim milk. Slice of angel food cake, store-bought or made from mix (from 10- or 11-inch-diameter cake, slice is 2 inches wide on the outside edge of cake). Top cake slice with one-half cup unsweetened fresh or frozen (thawed) strawberries or sliced peaches with juice (mash fruit lightly before pouring on cake). Cup of skim milk. Total, about 470 calories, 24 grams protein, 1 gram fat, 92 grams carbohydrate, 900 mg sodium, 24 mg cholesterol, 3 percent fat.

Reminders

■ Coffee, tea or diet pop are optional with all meals, but limit caffeine intake to two cups coffee or tea or four 12-ounce cola beverages per day (you may want to eliminate diet pop; research shows aspartame can stimulate appetites).
■ Two 80-calorie snacks are allowed per day. Use extra snacks or adjust meal portion sizes to achieve a daily calorie count that's right for your target weight (multiply target weight by 10; but if you're hungry, eat more of the legal snacks).
■ Don't forget to exercise.

9

*Week IV
of the
Dee-troit
Diet*

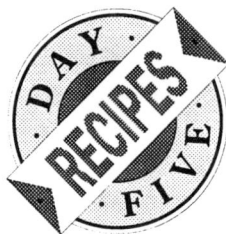

Seafood Kebab (a.k.a. "Fish Kebab")
(prepare ahead for Day 5 dinner)

1   cup lime juice, fresh or bottled
¼   cup onions, finely chopped
¼   teaspoon salt (optional)
     Dash of cayenne
½   pound fresh sea scallops (about 12 scallops)
1   sweet pepper (green, red or yellow)
1   medium zucchini, cut into ½-inch slices
4   Italian tomatoes, cut into ½-inch slices
8   large fresh mushrooms
4   shish kebab skewers, or other thin skewers
     at least 8 inches long

Mix lime juice, onions, salt and cayenne. Place scallops in a small glass or ceramic bowl. Pour lime juice mixture over scallops. Cover and place in refrigerator for at least 8 hours, preferably overnight.

After marinating, place on each skewer 1 scallop followed by single pieces of pepper, zucchini, tomato and a whole mushroom, repeating pattern until skewers are filled. Grill over coals or broil in oven. Do not overcook; after marinating in lime juice, scallops require only browning. Check often, turning a quarter turn every 2 minutes. Total broiling time is about 10 minutes. Serve with wedge of fresh lemon.

Serves four.

■ **Nutritional details per serving:** about 102 calories, 10 grams protein, trace of fat, 15 grams carbohydrate, 280 mg sodium, 20 cholesterol, 5 percent fat.

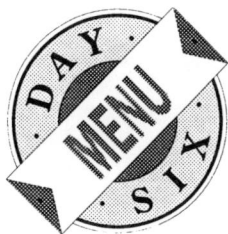

These are approximate nutritional totals for Day 6, averaging Breakfast A and B, but not including two 80-calorie snacks (see below): about 1,220 calories, 93 grams protein, 14 grams fat, 192 grams carbohydrate, 1,450 mg sodium, 165 mg cholesterol, 10 percent fat.

Breakfast

Choose A, B or C from Day 2, or choose any breakfast from the Substitute Breakfast page in the Appendix.

Lunch

Tuna sandwich: Mix 3½ ounces (half a small can) of water-packed tuna (preferably low-salt type) with 2 tablespoons of low-fat cottage cheese (1-percent milkfat only) and 1 tablespoon of chopped celery (optional: add 1 tablespoon chopped green onion). Serve between 2 slices of whole wheat bread; or add several lettuce leaves and stuff inside the halves of 1 whole round of pita bread (6-inch diameter). Whole fresh fruit. Cup of skim milk. Total: about 436 calories, 43 grams protein, 3 grams fat, 59 grams carbohydrate, 550 mg sodium, 69 mg cholesterol, 6 percent fat.

Dinner

Near Burger 'n' Near Beer night: Turkey Burger Deluxe (recipe follows), served with several lettuce leaves and ½ tomato, sliced. One-half ounce pretzels (one 8-inch-by-½-inch diameter log or about 4 three-ring pretzels; low-salt types are available). Two large sweet pickle spears ("bread and butter" pickles), or equivalent amount of small or sliced pickles. One 12-ounce non-alcoholic malt beverage such as Heileman's Kingsbury, Guinness Kaliber or Clausthaler (serve malt beverage VERY cold). Whole fresh fruit. Total, about 520 calories, 33 grams protein, 9 grams fat, 85 grams carbohydrate, 625 mg sodium, 88

9

*Week IV
of the
Dee-troit
Diet*

mg cholesterol, 15 percent fat.

(Note: a second malt beverage adds only 60 calories, no fat and lots of filling carbonation.)

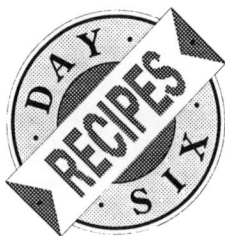

Turkey Burger Deluxe

½ teaspoon or 1 packet beef bouillon crystals
  (preferably low-sodium type)
2 tablespoons warm water

Per burger:
¼ pound ground turkey (buy fresh, skinless
  ground turkey; frozen ground turkey tends
  to be much higher in fat; place ground turkey
  in freezer if you are not planning to use it
  within a day or two)
¼ cup chopped onion
¼ cup chopped mushrooms
¼ teaspoon Mrs. Dash Salt-Free seasoning
  (regular)

Dissolve bouillon crystals in water and set aside. Mix turkey with onion and mushrooms, squeezing vegetables throughout meat. Shape into burger patty, and cook in non-stick skillet, wiped lightly with vegetable oil, over medium heat for about 5 minutes on each side. Remove burger from skillet temporarily and pour bouillon mixture in. Immediately replace burger and allow to simmer in bouillon juice, turning once or twice to absorb bouillon. Allow to cook several additional minutes per side. Do not undercook ("rare" turkey burger is a no-no). Serve in a hamburger bun (try Wonder Light buns — less fat and only 80 calories); with your choice of lettuce, tomato slices, mustard, relish, catsup.

■ **Nutrition details per burger and bun:** 300 calories, 31 grams protein, 8 grams fat, 27 grams carbohydrate, 300 mg sodium, 88 mg cholesterol, 22 percent fat.

9

*Week IV
of the
Dee-troit
Diet*

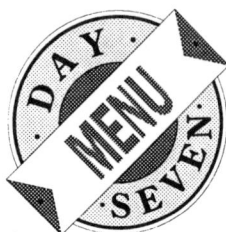

These are approximate nutritional totals for Day 7, averaging breakfast choices and using Lunch A, but not including two 80-calorie snacks (see below): about 1,210 calories, 61 grams protein, 11 grams fat, 223 grams carbohydrate, 1,560 mg sodium, 72 mg cholesterol, 8 percent fat.

Breakfast

Choose A, B or C from Day 2, or choose any breakfast from the Substitute Breakfast page in the Appendix.

Lunch

A. Bagel and yogurt lunch. Plain, garlic or whole-wheat bagel (or 2 slices whole wheat bread or toast); spread with 1-2 tablespoons low-sugar jam or jelly. One cup low-sugar low-fat fruit yogurt (no more than about 200 calories and 4 grams fat, such as the Dannon "25 percent less sugar" brands). Medium-size fresh carrot and stalk celery, cut into strips. Total: about 440 calories, 17 grams protein, 5 grams fat, 86 grams carbohydrate, 540 mg sodium, 14 mg cholesterol, 10 percent fat.

B. Soup lunch: 12-ounce bowl of non-cream meatless vegetable or tomato soup (preferably low-salt type; check label: no more than 2 grams of fat per serving). Two slices of bread, preferably whole wheat (or 1 bagel) with 2 tablespoons low-sugar jam or jelly; whole piece of fruit or sliced fruit plate without dressing. Scoop of orange or lemon sherbet (quarter cup; 70-calorie serving). Cup of skim milk. Total: about 500 calories, 18 grams protein, 6 grams fat, 94 grams carbohydrates, 1,718 mg sodium, 4 mg cholesterol, 11 percent fat.

Dinner

Serving of Gourmet Chicken and Fresh Vegetables (recipe follows).

Two slices toast or low-fat dinner roll (preferably whole wheat; served without butter). Whole piece of fresh fruit (or 1 cup sliced mixed fruit). Slice of angel food cake, store-bought or made from mix (from 10- or 11-inch-diameter cake, slice is 2 inches wide on the edge of cake), prepared as Chocolate Layered Angel Food Cake (recipe follows). Total, about 500 calories, 29 grams protein, 4 grams fat, 89 grams carbohydrate, 740 mg sodium, 44 mg cholesterol, 7 percent fat.

Reminders

■ Coffee, tea or diet pop are optional with all meals, but limit caffeine intake to two cups coffee or tea or four 12-ounce cola beverages per day (you may want to eliminate diet pop; research shows aspartame can stimulate appetites).

■ Two 80-calorie snacks are allowed per day. Use extra snacks or adjust meal portion sizes to achieve a daily calorie count that's right for your target weight (multiply target weight by 10; but if you're hungry, eat more of the legal snacks).

■ Don't forget to exercise.

9

Week IV
of the
Dee-troit
Diet

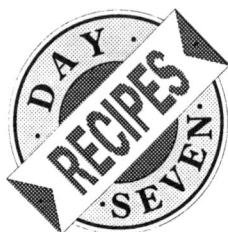

Gourmet Chicken and Fresh Vegetables

1   cup snow peas, with ends trimmed off
1   medium zucchini, thinly sliced
½   green pepper, cut in ½-inch pieces
½   red pepper, cut in ½-inch pieces (remove
    seeds and membrane from both peppers)
1   cup broccoli florets (large stalks trimmed
    off)
2   stalks celery, finely sliced
3   green onions, chopped
1   carrot, sliced
1   cup bean sprouts (optional — but a fine
    addition)
½   pound cooked skinless chicken
1   cup seasoned rice vinegar
1   tablespoon orange juice concentrate, if de-
    sired

Place in large bowl all vegetables. (Except for onions, you should have about 1 cup of each vegetable; peppers combine to make 1 cup.) Tear chicken into pieces and add. For tangy salad, toss with 1 cup seasoned rice vinegar (such as Marukan Seasoned Gourmet Rice Vinegar). For sweeter salad, combine vinegar with 1 tablespoon orange juice concentrate before tossing.

Serves four.

■ **Nutrition details per serving:** about 150 calories, 20 grams protein, 2 grams fat, 13 grams carbohydrate, 320 mg sodium, 44 mg cholesterol, 12 percent fat.

Chocolate Layered Angel Food Cake

1   5-ounce box, Jell-O Cook 'n Serve Pudding
     & Pie Filling
3   cups skim or ½-percent milk
1   unfrosted angel food cake (from mix, recipe
     or store-bought; 10-to-11-inch diameter
     cake)

Prepare pudding according to package directions, using skim or ½-percent milk (don't use whole milk). After pudding has chilled, slice cake 3 times horizontally so there are 4 cake layers. Using about 1 cup of pudding, spread pudding between cake layers and on top of cake. Serve in slices about 2 inches wide on outside edge.

■ **Nutrition details per slice:** about 150 calories, 3 grams protein, trace of fat, 35 grams carbohydrate, 100 mg sodium, 0 mg cholesterol, 1 percent fat.

The Body Mechanics

*So long — and welcome
to the rest of your life ...
And keep the Dee-troit Diet
in mind, too. It's your start
to a lifetime of enjoying
tasty, low-fat foods and
recipes.*

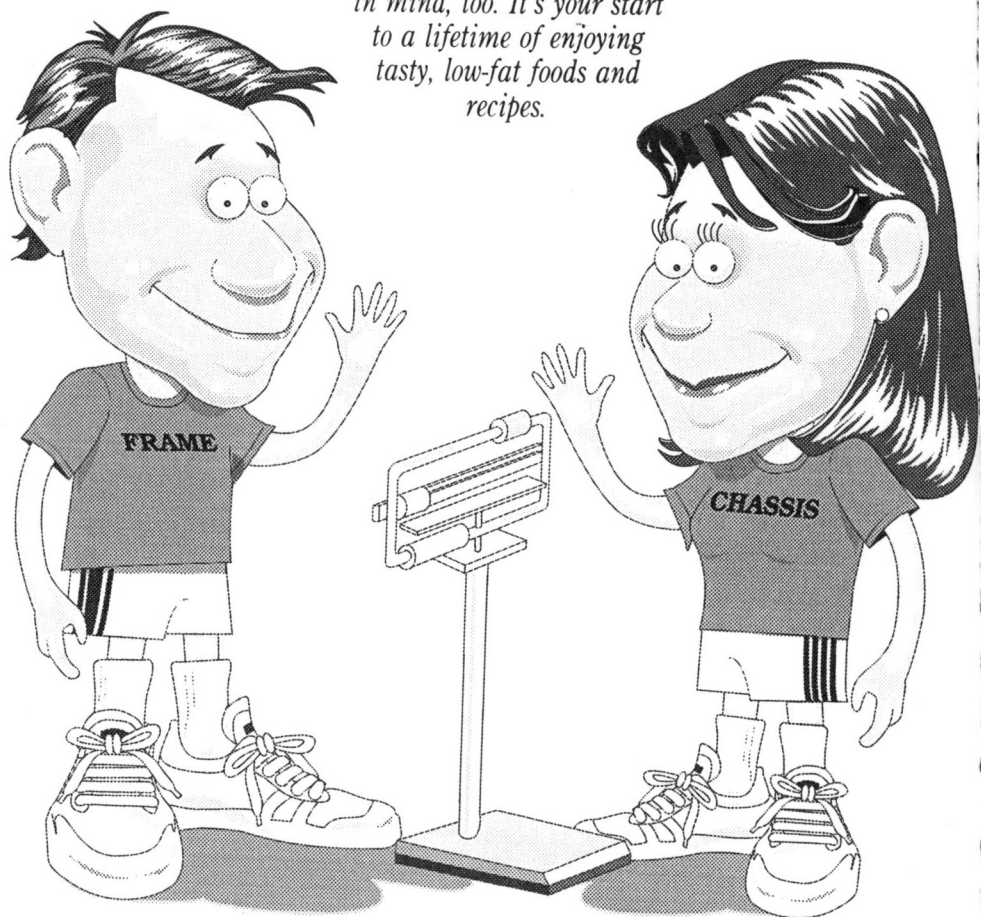

Appendix I:
Substitute Breakfasts

You can substitute any of the following for breakfasts listed in this book's menu plans.

Optional with all are coffee, tea or diet pop. If you normally add cream, whole milk or non-dairy coffee creamer to your coffee or tea, use skim milk instead.

To avoid excess caffeine, limit coffee or strong tea to two cups daily, and 12-ounce diet cola beverages to four per day. You may want to eliminate diet pop, however; research shows aspartame can stimulate appetites.

Where breakfasts call for "one whole fresh fruit" you can substitute half a grapefruit or half a cup mixed fresh fruit slices.

1. FRENCH TOAST: Two slices whole-wheat toast, dipped in mixture of one egg white beaten (optional: mix in 1-2 tablespoons oat bran). Brown both sides in non-stick pan sprayed with cooking spray. Top with one cup sliced fresh fruit.

Cup of skim milk or cup of plain non-fat yogurt. Optional: 2 tablespoons low-sugar maple syrup, or low-sugar jam or jelly, for toast.

2. OATMEAL: Hot bowl of oatmeal (⅓-½ cup, uncooked). (Optional: mix in 1-2 tablespoons oat bran.) Top with cup of skim milk or plain non-fat yogurt. Pour over oatmeal 1 cup sliced fresh fruit; or eat separately one whole orange or other fresh fruit.

3. MUFFIN/BAGEL AND YOGURT: One English muffin or bagel (preferably whole wheat); spread with 1-2 tablespoons low-sugar jam or or jelly. Cup of sliced fresh fruit poured over 1 cup of plain non-fat yogurt.

4. PANCAKES: Two 6-inch pancakes made from pancake mix, using skim milk and egg whites or low-fat egg substitute such as Egg Beaters (optional: mix in 1-2 tablespoons oat bran). Cook in non-stick pan sprayed lightly with cooking spray. Top with low-sugar maple syrup, or low-sugar jam or jelly.

One piece of whole fresh fruit (or pour over pancakes one cup sliced fresh fruit). Cup of skim milk.

5. TOAST AND YOGURT: One cup sliced fresh fruit, poured over one cup plain non-fat yogurt. Two slices of bread (preferably whole wheat), toasted, spread with 1-2 tablespoons low-sugar jam or jelly.

6. MUFFIN: Oat bran muffin (see Day 2 Menu in Chapter Nine for how to use a Duncan Hines mix). One cup plain non-fat yogurt topped with one cup sliced fresh fruit; or cup of skim milk and one whole piece of fresh fruit.

Appendix II:
For More Information . . .

To make Dee-troit Dieting a lifetime habit, seek out other sources of nutrition advice and low-fat recipes. Cooking Light magazine, available in many book and magazine stores, is an excellent source.

There are many fine books. Some contain a few recipes and many general cooking suggestions; others are mainly recipes. Here are a few of our favorites:

■ "8-Week Cholesterol Cure Cookbook," Harper & Row, $19.95.

■ "Menu for Life" by Joan Klun Kaye and L.E. Smith, Menu For Life Inc., $14.95, plus tax and $2.50 shipping for a total of $18.15; to order by Visa or Mastercard, call 313-375-2130 in Rochester, Mich., 9-5 weekdays.

■ "Eater's Choice — A Food Lover's Guide To Lower Cholesterol" by Dr. Ron Goor and Nancy Goor, Houghton Mifflin Co., $11.95 paperback.

■ "Eat Fish, Live Better" by Anne Fletcher, Harper & Row, $18.95.

■ "The New American Diet" by Sonja Connor and Dr. William Connor, Simon & Schuster, $12.95 paperback.

■ "Lose Weight Naturally" by Mark Bricklin, Rodale Press Books, $24.95.

And for help with the psychological side of obesity, we found a lot to like in the following:

■ "Weight, Sex & Marriage — A Delicate Balance" by Richard Stuart and Barbara Jacobson, Fireside Books, $6.95 paperback.

■ "Overcoming Overeating" by Jane Hirschmann and Carol Munter, Fawcett/Columbine, $8.95 paperback.

■ "Making Peace with Food" by Susan Kano, Harper & Row, $10.95.